HOW TO CURE AND PREVENT ANY DISEASE

FIVE EASY WAYS YOU CAN ENJOY VIBRANT HEALTH, HAPPINESS AND LONGEVITY

BY RAY GEBAUER

(www.cureanydisease.com)

Published by Freedom Unlimited, Inc.
15000 SE 38th St. #800
Bellevue, WA 98006

Publisher's Cataloging-in Publication Data
Gebauer, Ray
    How to cure and prevent any disease: five easy ways you can enjoy vibrant health, happiness and longevity / Ray Gebauer – Bellevue, WA: Freedom Unlimited, Inc., 2000.
        p.   cm.
    ISBN 0-9674782-0-0

    1. Medicine, Preventive. 2. Health. I. Title.
RA776 .G43 2000   99-66754
613--dc21   CIP

PROJECT COORDINATION BY JENKINS GROUP, INC.

02 01 00 99 ▲ 5 4 3 2 1

Printed in the United States of America

Praise for

How to Cure and Prevent Any Disease

"An excellent, well-written practical resource. If you care about your state of health, you will want to read Ray Gebauer's "How To Cure and Prevent Any Disease."

Blaine S. Purcell, M.D., Diplomate, American Board of Internal Medicine and American Board of Anti-Aging Medicine

---

"It is difficult in a few words to convey the importance of the concepts that Ray Gebauer has presented in this remarkable book. I have been on the front lines of the war against disease and illness and can tell you that we have been losing the battle utilizing the acute interventive approach to health and disease. I know this all too well personally, having lost my mother to lung cancer in 1980, and nearly 20 years later, lost my father-in-law from the very same cancer. What was remarkable is that the treatment and prognosis over that 20-year span barely changed. We are however in the midst of an incredible change. Rarely do we perceive a revolution like that presented here.

"The biggest revolutionary change is represented by glyconutrients, taking its place as one of the pivotal classes of nutrients supporting human health. I know this not only because of the medical studies but also by the profound effects it has had toward promoting health in my patients that had been lacking over the past 20 years. If you do not want to become a patient (and therefore a statistic) you need to answer in your own mind and heart if what you are doing for your health is optimal, and if not what else can you do. This book offers that path to optimal health."

Michael D. Schlachter, MD, Board Certified Internal Medicine and Pulmonary Disease Clinical Instructor, University of Nevada Medical School

"A superb, timely and practical book that has been needed for a long time. I personally would not be a physician today if I had not utilized glyconutrients. They have revolutionized the health care field. The time is here for us all to take responsibility for our health. Treating symptoms has had it's day. Thank you Ray for your contributions."

Eleanor L.M. Dubey, D.C., Ph.D.

"Your book, "How to Cure and Prevent Any Disease" is truly remarkable and fascinating. Insights are offered to enjoy a more rewarding and satisfying life that good health can bring. My own battle with cancer would have been much easier and much less frightening with this information. Thank you, Ray, for your contribution to the thousands of people who will benefit."

Michael A. Currieri, Ph.D. Diplomate in Neurotherapy Certified QEEGT Certified EEG Biofeedback Provider

---

"My father once said to my brother and I, " If you want to know the answer, ask the man who knows." Ray Gebauer is a man who knows. He is always finding innovative and exciting ways to share his knowledge with those around him. Ray is a seemingly common man with an amazingly uncommon vision of helping hundreds of thousands of people improve their health as well as their wealth. God has blessed him with the gifts of help and discernment as well as giving. Rays' new book will be a tremendous help and blessing to those who read it and use it in their lives and businesses, and should be a mandatory addition to your library."

Stanley C. Allison, MD, Diplomate of the American Board of Ophthalmology Certified Diabetes Educator, Tacoma, Washington

---

"At last someone has written a book explaining the scientific principles of preventive health-care in a simple and easy to understand format. I have been teaching the biblical principles of health and doing private nutritional counseling for over 35 years, and now I can recommend a book that brings the pieces of the puzzle together! I especially appreciate how Ray shows that

the new scientific discoveries in health care gives God, not man, the glory.

"In the future, many books and scientific studies will be written about "glyconutritionals." However, we can understand the importance of their discovery in the here-and-now because Ray's book is written in a down-to-earth fashion that anyone can understand. Good health cannot help but come to those who truly apply the principles of this book to their lives. Everyone needs this book!"

Ken Anderson, Nutritional Consultant for 35 years, former Health Resort Owner, Oregon

---

"We are all beginning to realize that responsibility for optimal health lies with each of us, and not with a doctor. But where do you go to learn how to take responsibility for your health? This outstanding book, How To Prevent and Cure Any Disease, shows you how to take back this responsibility and your health!

"You will learn that there are a number of very effective strategies to regaining control of your own health. Throughout this text, you will discover the integration of science and your "natural" self, allowing you to own the decision-process. The majority of Americans are looking for this balanced individual approach, but not knowing where to find it. Well, here it is. I believe that this book can make a very significant difference for thousands of people across this country and around the world. Thank you, Ray, for this invaluable contribution."

Dr. Steven M. Hines, O.D., BS in Microbiology, emphasis in Immunology, BS in Zoology, emphasis in Biochemistry and Physiology, BS in Visual Science and Neuro-physiology, Diplomate in Vision Therapy and Sports Vision, Woodinville, Washington

---

"How to Cure and Prevent Any Disease" by Ray Gebauer is both inspiring and enlightening - a sure-fire combination to educate the masses. Highly recommended.

Ann Louise Gittleman, M.S., C.N.S., Author of <u>Your Body Knows Best</u>

Dedication

To Diana, my beloved wife, the light of my life,
and to God my Father who is my life.

Table of Contents

Appendixes

Preface

Imagine yourself sitting in an airplane listening to the routine instructions of what to do if there were an emergency. What kind of attention would you be giving to this? If you've heard this dozens of times as I have, you may, as most people appear to do, give this very little serious attention.

Let's suppose that half way through the flight the stewardess stood up and began to repeat the safety instructions, but this time prefaced the routine with this statement.

"Folks, may I have your attention. Due to a mechanical malfunction, this plane is going down. I am going to repeat the instructions I gave at the beginning of the flight. If you follow the instructions completely, you have a 99 percent chance of survival. If you don't, you have a 95 percent chance of not surviving."

Now, given this context, how much attention would you be giving to the safety instructions? It would be a little different this time, wouldn't it?

This is exactly how I am requesting you give your attention to what you are about to read, because it is just as serious as in this example. *Unless people start doing certain things differently, 95 percent of the population "is going down" and will not survive the current health disaster that will be fully explained in the next few pages. If you give this information your full attention and act on it, you are far more likely to be in the surviving 5 percent.*

My Gift to You

This book is not just about giving you some new or interesting information. *It's my gift to you—a gift of life.*

This is a gift that gives you a way to escape being in that 95 percent category (the health disaster).

This is a gift that gives you strategies that you can actually use to cure and prevent any disease.

This is a gift that gives you ways to experience vibrant health, happiness and longevity. The seventy-seven true stories of real people are included as evidence to show that it *is actually possible* to cure diseases, rather than this just being some theory. They are meant as real life illustrations of how the body can overcome disease and heal itself.

This may be one of the most important books you've read in your life, but it will be worth absolutely nothing to you if you don't take it seriously, and if you don't alter your perspective and lifestyle. You can't afford the exorbitant cost of staying stuck in your old ways! And you don't want to go where it's taking you!

My purpose in writing this book is two-fold. I wanted to create a vehicle that could be used to literally save and change the lives of people around the world. For that reason, this book is an important part of fulfilling my destiny of making a significant difference for people. I know what it feels like to save the life of just one person. The possibility of saving and enriching the lives of millions is awesome!

The "Midas Touch"

My second purpose in writing this book is to give you another kind of gift—the gift of the "Midas Touch." In the story of King Midas, he was given the power to turn everything he touched to gold. As you know, this gift became a curse, because it was used solely out of greed.

This book can give you a different kind of "Midas Touch." This is the "Midas touch of health" which is the knowledge of how to help people regain their health, which is even more precious than gold.

This gift is for you and for thousands of other caring people like you so that you can touch the lives of the people you care most about, and as a result, we can collectively impact the lives of *millions* of people across the world.

Some people have as their mission to save the earth and its environment. This certainly is indeed a worthy, noble and necessary goal, and I'm grateful people are putting attention on that.

My mission is to play my role in saving and enriching the lives of its inhabitants. I identify with the words of the ancient prophet Isaiah from 2700 years ago:

"...bring good news to the afflicted; ... bind up the broken-hearted, proclaim freedom to captives...and announce a time of healing (grace)."

I sincerely invite you to join me in this health freedom crusade. Millions of lives are at stake in the areas of physical, emotional and spiritual health. Whose lives? Yours and at least 95 percent of the people you know. Who you are and what you do really can make an important difference.

Plus it is only in enriching the lives of others that our own lives are enriched.

My hope for you is that through this book, you will find the reasons and pathway to be a part of this crusade to enrich the lives of others. Your reward can be spectacular, as mine has already been! Thank you.

Acknowledgements

I appreciate each of the hundreds of people who have invested deliberately and unconsciously in my personal growth and in my life. Who I am, the position I am in and the impact I can make is only because of how others have given and contributed to my life.

I appreciate the many mentors in my life starting with Kenneth Prickett, who became a sort of substitute father for seven years starting in the fifth grade; Jim Rohn, my philosophical teacher and success coach in life; John Wimber, Mike Bickle, Jack Deere and Rick Joyner for the examples their lives are of passion for God; Larry Crabb and John Piper, the two authors who gave me the greatest insight into life; and Mike Smith, for helping me break out of most of my intellectualism and self-righteousness and showing me how to coach and empower others.

I appreciate Sam Caster and the many leaders and associates in Mannatech who are part of the mission to make a difference in this world.

I especially appreciate my extraordinary wife, Diana—I am so proud of her and love her with all my heart.

Most of all, I appreciate God my Father for the lavish grace and blessings He has given me. They are far beyond what I could ever deserve. He is Awesome!

God is good!
God is great!
And I am grateful!

Foreword

I am writing this forward from inside the triple fortifications of the ancient Castle of Carcassonne in Southeastern France. It exemplifies the concepts of this excellent and timely book by Ray Gebauer in several important ways.

This book is one of the most important sources that you may ever read, for it will provide you with scientifically verified concepts that demonstrate how to *fortify* your own body in order to prevent the onset of diseases in you or one of your loved ones. You will also learn how you can *re-fortify* when one of these diseases strike so as to stop the attack and in most cases reverse much or all of the damage. I hope my analogy of the ancient fortification of Carcassonne will help introduce you to these concepts.

Initially, this magnificent edifice began as a *cathedral*, a place built for the glory of God. Its birth was almost a millenium ago in 1096.

Like a newborn baby, it was not only a work of God, but also like a newborn, was scantly protected from the harsh elements. Its defenses were weak.

A newborn baby is most susceptible to sickness at birth because the immune system is not fully developed. Mother's milk has been uniquely designed to fortify a baby's defenses at this time. As such, breast-feeding is one of the most important contributions a mother can provide to protect her baby and begin the process of fortifying the baby's immune system so that it can protect itself from diseases.

(There is also hope for those mothers who cannot breast feed—the most important protective element in mother's milk has been uncovered by science—glyconutrients, or essential saccharides [carbohydrates] which will be discussed later in this book.)

But the cathedral needed more solid defenses. The FIRST

protective wall was constructed in the 12th Century, which resulted in a castle. It was solid enough to protect a small force of Cathars (a sect of Christians interested in living a particularly pure life, insulated from the corrupted politics of the time) against a "holy" crusade, consisting of a large army of northern barons and their knights led by Simon de Montfort. The leader of the Cathars, Raymond-Roger Trencavel used a concept (protection by fortification) that this book will explain.

Think of the cathedral inside of the castle as your body and the northern barons, the enemy, as viruses, bacteria, toxins, pollutants, food contaminants and other environmental factors that are DAILY conspiring to rob you of your health and your life. Prior to the building of the castle walls, the area surrounding the cathedral was NOT enough to protect the Cathars who occupied the cathedral. This castle wall provided necessary protection, which in your body would include fortification by using the five strategies presented in this book. Consider using the essential nutrients also suggested in this book to protect yourself as the Cathars did.

Incidentally, the downfall of the Cathars was due to not having enough water. This same lack also can be a critical factor in the breakdown of the physical body.

Later, the Castle fell into the hands of Saint Louis, king of France. He built a SECOND set of walls around the castle to strengthen it even further. Now further fortified, the castle was able to withstand a large number of assaults and sieges. The construction of the outer defenses had more than doubled the protection of the defense works. The king understood an important concept—the stronger your castle, the more attacks it can withstand, thus creating more security.

The same goes for our body. We live in a harsh, polluted environment crawling with uncountable microorganisms. These forces continually attempt to invade your castle, the body, and conspire to make you sick or even cause your death. Infections like malaria, pneumonia, diarrheal illnesses, AIDS, tuberculosis and hepatitis viruses still account for millions of deaths worldwide each year, especially in the countries with the weakest defenses—third world nations with extremely poor nutrition.

However, in developed countries, we are not immune to diseases of the environment either! Viruses and poor nutrition have been linked with leading killers like heart disease, cancer and diabetes, which are on the rise each year! As our planet is becoming more polluted and toxic, we need to fortify our personal castles using every resource we can.

Later, kings of France added a THIRD set of walls! And this leads to the modern Castle of Carcassonne, which acted as the primary bastion of defense from attacks coming from the South for over six centuries! As military art had evolved and had reached its pinnacle in defensive fortifications, so is science now reaching such a point in the art of health defense and dietary supplementation, as this book so brilliantly illustrates.

Eventually, as our body ages, it sometimes needs to be rebuilt despite our best efforts at defense. In 1853, the castle was in dire need of repairs. Eugene Viollet-le-Duc made it his life's work to rebuild the castle. Despite the considerable historical importance of this castle (and your health!), it was a fight to find the funding for its restoration (even today, people struggle to find funding for their own health restoration). The government, lead by Napolean III, attempted to interfere by cutting off funding. But Viollet-le-Duc and his underwriters were PERSISTENT. They believed that this important structure must be restored, and were able to creatively find the necessary funding as sometimes we need to do for our own health maintenance and restoration.

The castle was completely restored by the 1870's, and still stands in magnificence today. It is the best maintained of all castles dating back that far in history despite the many wars, sieges and ravages of time it withstood over the centuries.

The reasons that this spectacular monument, representative of our bodies, is still standing and well maintained are multifold:

It was protected from an early age
Over time, its fortifications were reinforced and enhanced
When it began to crumble, it was repaired
The science behind its defenses and repair was the very best

The defenses and restoration of the Castle used five natural resources— fire, earth, metal (rock and sand), water, wood, plus ingenuity.

Nothing artificial was used. Everything contributed to its defense instead of merely "masking weaknesses" like most drugs do. Making the castle simply look better (Perhaps an equivalent would be the use of drugs to merely make you feel better!) would not have allowed it to stand to this day!

Two thousand years before this cathedral was built, an ancient prophet wrote these words:

"A man without self-control is like a defenseless city without walls that is easily broken into." Proverbs 25:28

This book will enable you to discover for yourself how best to defend, fortify and repair your Castle. In view of the value of your health and life, that is certainly a worthwhile project!

I found this book to be accurate and most informative. Using the advice contained within the following pages, you will be best prepared to live a long, healthful life. Because there is too much at stake (people's lives) to keep this invaluable information to yourself, please share it with others as well!

Thank you for doing everything you can to help others discover how they can have vibrant health and longevity. Equipped with this information, perhaps you can be a hero to someone whose castle is in need of fortification and repair.

DARRYL SEE, MD
Associate Clinical Professor of Medicine
World Health Organization
Director of the Institute of Longevity Medicine
Director, Bioassay Laboratory
Co-chair of Research, American Nutraceutical Association

Introduction
THE SHOCKING TRUTH
NO ONE'S TALKING ABOUT

Is it really possible to cure or prevent disease, or is this just hype to get your attention? Based on the evidence in thousands of people's lives, as well as my personal observations, it is *absolutely* possible to prevent and/or cure all diseases and to enjoy vibrant health, happiness and longevity. Seventy-seven true stories of real people are included to help you believe that this really is possible.

In this book, you will learn how you can do this. Plus, you'll learn how you can help other people do this also.

Everything in life has both a payoff and a price. Living without regard to your health has the short-term payoff of a false sense of freedom. Sooner or later you pay a terrible price for your indifference, ignorance or negligence. The wiser alternative is to pay the price up front in diligence and discipline and enjoy the payoff of vibrant health for the rest of your life. You either pay now or pay later—so why not pay the smaller cost up front and enjoy the greater benefit for the longer term?

Most people will spend more money to insure their house or car, which are replaceable, than they do on their health, which is not replaceable! If your house burns down or your car wears out, you can always get a new one; not so with your body.

Where are you going to live when your body wears out?

Three thousand years ago, the prophet Hosea said, *"My people perish for lack of knowledge."* Can you see how this is still true today? Millions of people are dying each year simply because they lack the critical knowledge that could have preserved their health.

The World Health Organization has identified the two major obstacles in modern society to enjoying vibrant health and longevity: ignorance and complacency.

Ignorance and complacency are the two most serious threats to your health, happiness and longevity.

Ignorance is just a lack of knowledge, but complacency is based on false assumptions, such as "everything is okay for me—I'm healthy." Ignorance and complacency are your most dangerous enemies, and unfortunately they have the vast financial reinforcement from huge corporations that virtually brainwash us and our children through incessant advertising that perpetuates this problem.

In light of this, you have a tremendous opportunity to make a significant difference for not only yourself and loved ones but for millions of people simply by sharing the concepts you will be discovering in this book.

In fact, the World Health Organization is mounting a major campaign to battle these two public health enemies. Three thousand years earlier, another authority, King Solomon put it this way: *"The drifting along of simple minded (naïve) people shall kill them, and the complacency of fools will destroy them."* Proverbs 1:32. You can be a part of this crusade against ignorance and complacency and be a part in saving lives!

Seeing clearly the seriousness of the problem AND what is at stake is the only way to have an ongoing motivation to do something about it. So really, just how bad is the health crisis?

95 PERCENT IS OBSCENE!

Here are the facts—judge for yourself! Over 50 percent of Americans will die from heart or vascular disease (including strokes); 33 percent will die from cancer; and 12 percent will die from diabetes. What do these top three causes of death add up to? An **obscene 95 percent!** That's just the top three!

A century ago, probably less than 5 percent of Americans died from these diseases! Now it's common place. Most people *expect* to have aches and pains, high blood pressure, tiredness, heart problems, and other common place degenerative diseases when they get older. Why? Because about everyone else develops these, so it seems normal.

In 1996, according to the Center for Disease Control, 894,265 people died from heart/vascular disease and 544,278 people died from cancer. That's almost 4,000 people a day, or *one death every twenty-two seconds!* Each year the numbers are higher.

Living in the Health Disaster Zone

This is a health disaster of unimaginable proportions! We are living in an unprecedented *health disaster zone.*

As if this were not bad enough, the experts are predicting that other types of health disasters are coming. *U.S. News & World Report* warns that a world wide epidemic of Hepatitis C is imminent and inevitable. According to an article in the February 1998 issue of *Time* magazine, this next *pandemic* is expected to kill 60 million people worldwide, and we have *no* drugs or antibiotics to help against this coming health disaster.

Death by Prescription

What would you guess is the *fourth* leading cause of death? According to the American Medical Association, it is from the well-intentioned efforts to *recover* health: prescription drugs! Over 200,000 people a year die from "adverse reactions" from drugs, and another 80,000 die from medical malpractice, whereas 41,000 die in auto accidents, according to the pharmacy industry magazine, <u>Drug Topics</u>, October 23, 1995, pg. 14-16! *That's one death every two minutes!*

Here's another way of looking at it. You have a seven times greater chance of dying walking into your doctor's office than you do getting behind the wheel of your car!

This is from the *legal* drugs prescribed by doctors to people trying to manage their pain and symptoms (only 20,000 die as a result of illegal drug use)! An additional two million people suffer some sort of injury!

It's common knowledge that *100 percent of drugs are toxic. There is no safe drug.* Yet *Americans spend over eleven million dollars a day on drugs!* By definition and law, a drug must have a measurable toxic level that is lethal. So, while drugs do have their place, perhaps you should keep them in the proper place (last) and consider drugs to be your *last* resort, not your *first* resort!

The Illusion of Protection

Don't make the mistake of thinking that just because the FDA has approved of a drug or procedure, or that your doctor prescribes it that it is safe. According to the General Accounting Office, 102 of the 198 drugs approved by the FDA between 1978 and 1986 had *"serious post-approval risks such as heart failure...convulsions...kidney and liver failure...birth defects and blindness."*

In fact, one food additive approved by the FDA is so dangerous, it was once classified by the Pentagon as a biochemical weapon!

The most common treatment for prostate problems, which 60 percent of men over 50 develop, is surgery. Of course this is approved by the FDA and is touted as a "safe procedure" by urologists. Yet one study found that a year after prostate surgery, 41percent of men had to wear diapers because of chronic leakage, and 88 percent were finished sexually because of total impotence!

Former FDA Commissioner, Dr. Herbert Ley stated, *"The thing that bugs me is that the people think the FDA is protecting them. It isn't. What the FDA is doing and what the public thinks it's doing are as different as night and day."*

For more information on the risk of using drugs, visit the eye opening web site, www.drugawareness.org.

What are you going to do?

The incontrovertible truth has been and always will be, that **if you do what most people do, you'll get what most people get!**

In light of the grim 95 percent statistic, that is not very comforting!

*What are you doing to make sure **you** are not part of the 95 percent category?*

As you can see, ignorance is NOT bliss! Whether it's ignorance, complacency or negligence, you'll get the same results: disease and premature death. Three thousand years later it's still true—*"people perish for lack of knowledge."*

If you want something different, you've got to be willing to do something different! *If you want vibrant health, happiness and longevity, you've got to do something different from what 95 percent of the population are doing.*

If you keep going in the same direction, you will end up where you are headed!

This book discusses five easy strategies to vibrant health, happiness and longevity so *you* will know what to do differently. You don't *have* to be a part of that appalling category! Rather than being a *victim*, you can actually be a *hero* by sharing what you learn with others so that they don't have to be a part of that unfortunate majority either!

To help you remember these five important strategies to vibrant health, happiness and longevity, I've arbitrarily associated them with the five dynamics in the Oriental Healing model: Fire, Earth, Metal, Water and Wood (no religious connections are intended).

Your Health Checking Account

One useful way to understand how health works is to use the

analogy of a checking account. As you know, deposits *increase* your balance and the checks you write *decrease* your balance. When the amount of the checks exceed the sum of your deposits, you get bounced checks!

The same thing occurs with your body. Everything you do that *contributes* to your health is a deposit. Any kind of stress (physical, mental, emotional, chemical, electromagnetic) is a "stress check" written against your account. When the amount of "stress checks" exceed the sum of your "deposits," you have "non-sufficient funds," which shows up as pain or as a health disorder and eventually as disease!

This analogy explains why some people who are clearly not doing healthy things for themselves do not have any major health breakdowns for years or decades. Because initially they have a high enough "balance" in their health account, they can keep writing checks for years before they have "Non-Sufficient Funds (NSF)." Very often, this is a genetic gift from their parents. But, if that "inherited wealth" is carelessly squandered, it is inevitable that they will hit the NSF stage sooner. You don't want to waste your inheritance do you?

What you will want to do, now that you understand this dynamic more clearly, is to deliberately make daily deposits and build up your health reserves. Then you must be conscious and careful how you "write checks" that *deplete* your health balance.

The "deposits" are the five strategies to vibrant health and longevity, and the "checks" or "withdrawals" are any form of stress, which includes neglect.

People underestimate the seriousness of stress. According to Doc Childre, founder of HeartMath and consultant to Fortune 100 companies on dealing with stress and increasing productivity, *"stress stimulates the perpetual release of the hormones adrenaline, noradrenaline and cortisol, which eventually sear the body like a constant drizzle of acid. If left unchecked, chronic stress can sicken and eventually kill us."*

As much as 80 percent of all disease in the U.S. is initiated or aggravated by emotional stress according to a Harvard University study.
(This does not include other sources of stress such as chemical
stress from pollutants).

A twenty-year study by the University of London School of
Medicine determined that unmanaged mental and emotional
reactions to stress are a *more dangerous risk factor for cancer and
heart disease than cigarette smoking or eating high cholesterol foods.*

Mice and the Electric Grid Experiment

There is another critical factor that even outweighs the amount
of the "stress check" (the intensity or severity of the stress), and
that is the *frequency* of the stress. For more than fifty years,
researchers have known that putting stress on an animal greatly
accelerates the aging process. When mice are placed on an electric grid with very mild shocks, they are unaffected *as long as they
were given enough time to recover from the stress of the shocks.* But if
these mild shocks are too frequent, the mice are not able to
recover from this harmless stress, and they die from old age within a few short days.

An autopsy reveals many signs of accelerated aging. Even
though each electric shock itself was harmless, *the accumulative
effect of frequent stress causes the body to just give up and die.* When
you don't have enough time to recover from a particular stress
before the next one comes, your reserves and "account balance"
in your health account is quickly depleted.

Avoiding the Time Bomb

Most people, when they start getting "bounced checks" in their
health account, do the best they know, which is to take the
traditional route and try to *manage or suppress* their pain and
symptoms with drugs and/or surgery. This may buy you a little
more time while the real problem is driven deeper into your
body, creating a virtual time bomb with a long fuse. The alter-

native is that you can rebuild and recover your health by making larger and more frequent "health deposits" and allow fewer "stress checks" — both of which are accomplished through the five strategies you will learn about in this book.

HEALTH ILLUSIONS

One of the most dangerous perceptions that must be addressed is the common *assumption and illusion* that a person is healthy as long as he/she feels good. Millions of people are faked out by the *appearance* of good health. Health is *not* the absence of disease, pain or symptoms. Symptoms are the *last and final* stage of a breakdown that has been in process for years or decades.

Your body was designed with numerous redundant (backup) systems. It has a remarkable ability to compensate for deficiencies and problems for years. It will always "borrow from Peter to pay Paul," that is until Peter is broke, too. Then "bankruptcy" (of your health) is unavoidable because you have bounced checks all over the place!

Here are some examples to illustrate this truth. Cancer takes five to thirty years to develop to the point that it is detectable. During that time you feel great, or at least okay, because your body has been compensating and utilizing your backup reserves. Then you get the shock of your life when your doctor happens to discover that you have breast, liver, colon, or prostate cancer.

You can't believe it! Yesterday you were healthy and today you have terminal cancer! No, you only *thought* you were healthy, because you mistakenly equated feeling good with health.

Michael Landon is a tragic and vivid example of this. He appeared on the Johnny Carson show and displayed his "healthy" body that had been diagnosed with cancer of the pancreas. He had less than 10 percent body fat and was the picture of health and fitness. He told the nation that he'd never felt better in his life and that he was going to beat this! Three months later he was dead.

Fitness is NOT Health

Don't make the mistake of confusing fitness with health! Strong muscles don't mean you are healthy or that you have a strong immune system. Everyday, people in good shape, including trained athletes, die from cancer and heart disease. Most of us are still faked out by the "picture" of health, the superficial outward appearance.

Two thousand years ago, Jesus warned us, "*Do not judge according to appearance....*" But we still tend to do just that, don't we?

In other more obvious areas, we know better. Only a naive person would assume that a used car with a good body is in good condition. We know that it's what's on the inside that counts. But due to a "*lack of knowledge*" in the health arena, we assume otherwise in the most important area, our health, not realizing that what we don't know can kill us!

Iceberg Ahead

Heart disease is another classic example of this. Heart disease takes thirty to forty years to develop. Did you know that autopsies revealed that over 95 percent of the fit young men (teenagers) who died in the Vietnam War had advanced hardening of the arteries? Even autopsies of young children killed in accidents reveal clogged arteries, which is the first stage of heart disease! Probably over 90 percent of grade school children have the beginning of heart disease, which won't manifest for thirty to forty years! Is that health?

Did you know that 50 percent of the time the very first indication of a heart problem is a FATAL heart attack? We are so shocked! Joe was so "healthy," and suddenly he dies of a heart attack. We are shocked because we, like Joe, were ASSUMING in our ignorance, that Joe was healthy because he didn't have any outward pain or symptoms. We assume we are strong and healthy, like the Titanic headed for the unseen iceberg. The reality is that Joe had not been healthy for years. But, because his body was compensating for the imbalances, he and everyone else assumed he was just fine.

Over 95 percent of people already suffer from poor health. It's just a matter of time before it's evident. In fact, one third of Americans already have a diagnosed chronic disease! It's inevitable, that UNLESS you do something *different* from the 95 percent who are doomed to die prematurely from just the top three causes, you will too. BUT, if you are willing to make a few simple changes, it is possible and almost inevitable that you too can turn things around and have your own "miracle" as seventy-seven people have shared their miracle in this book.

Are you ready to do something different? If not, you might as well turn the TV back on. Don't waste your time reading any further.

1

YOU ONLY GET WHAT YOU PUT ON PAPER!

How Free Do You Want to Be?

Exactly What Do You Want?

What About Your Doctor?

Miracle Stories

How Free Do You Want To Be?

How much do you value your freedom? Do you *treasure* it, or do you take it for granted? If you had to lose one freedom, which would be the last one you would be willing to give up?

For many people, it's health freedom—the freedom to *have* vibrant health and longevity, and freedom *from* sickness and disability.

You may have already lost a considerable portion of your health freedom. If you have, it is not too late to do something different to get it back. Or if you *appear* to be healthy, and if you are doing what 95 percent of Americans are doing, it's only a matter of time that the health problems brewing under the surface will manifest and you find yourself a victim of the big three killers, and lose your freedom to even be alive!

Now is the time to decide how free you want to be! If you are truly serious about having health freedom, it is imperative that you shift your perspective on health in such a way that *how* you think about health and *what* you do with it changes.

Just hoping you "stay healthy" or wishing you were healthy again is not going to make any difference. The first step is a clear unalterable decision that you are committed to your health freedom—either in maintaining it or restoring it.

And to strengthen that even further, make a commitment to help others discover the reality of health freedom as well. As an extra benefit to doing this, you will experience a deep satisfaction and fulfillment that only comes from contribution and service to others. As you help others reclaim their health freedom, you will have accelerated the process for yourself!

So honestly, just how free do you want to be? How much freedom do you want?

Exactly What Do You Want?

Start by making a COMPLETE list of *every* health disorder you have, from your scalp to your toes, including minor issues—anything that is less than vibrant health. Now restate each condition as you would describe it, if in that area you were in perfect health. In other words, describe it as a *goal* without using negative language, such as "no pain."

For example, your health goal for backaches could be "a strong and stable back so I could do...." Diabetes could be "normal blood sugar." Cancer of the liver could be "a healthy liver." Overweight could be "my ideal weight." Arthritis could be "normal and flexible joint function." Poor memory could be "excellent memory." *State it the way you want to be.*

Now rate your current overall health on a scale from zero to ten, with ten being vibrant health (the way you want to be).

Then, using the same scale, rate each of your current health concerns, with zero being the most severe and ten being no problem (i.e., vibrant health). Now transfer these exact numbers to your list of health goals for each condition.

For example, you may rate your overall health as a six. You may rate your bad headaches as a three; therefore the rating for your positive goal for that condition (e.g., head feels great) would also be a three, with the goal being a ten. *You always want to get up to a ten.*

If in your case, it seems hard to believe that it could be possible (getting up to a ten), start by considering it as a possibility. Once you are comfortable with that idea, muster up the faith to make your goal something less than a ten, such as a seven. Then if you achieve that, you will have faith to go all the way for the ten!

For example, if you have colon cancer, that's pretty serious. You may give that a rating as low as "one." Your health goal could be a "healthy normal colon." Your health goal of course is to get it back up to a ten.

Select the goals that are most important to you and list the top three or five on a three-by-five note card. Place a copy of it in several places where you can see it each day. *Every time you "make a deposit" into your health account, by using one of the strategies you will be learning, do it with the conscious purpose and intention of achieving your top three health goals, and getting up to a ten.*

Every thirty days review your list of health goals and rate each item again. Note in a journal any improvement you have seen from following the five strategies.

It is vitally important that you clearly picture in your mind what you *want* to attain (your health goal) rather than on what you want to avoid or alleviate (disease) because *you will tend to get or keep whatever you are focusing your attention on.*

Jacques D. Barth, of the Southern California Prevention and Research Center in Los Angeles, discovered in a study of 210 volunteers, that people who carried an ultrasound image of one of their major (healthy) arteries in their wallet and posted a copy of the picture on their refrigerator were more likely to reduce their risk factors for heart disease than those who saw images of the arteries just once. *Therefore, see yourself as healthy every time you do something for your health!*

Because your body works on the most urgent issues first, usually you will not see progress in all areas at the same time. But eventually, if you stand in faith and act in faith, it is possible for you to have a "ten" on each of your health goals as long as you do all you can as long as it takes.

Remember that all freedom has its price. Are you willing to pay the price for your health freedom? Keep asking yourself the question: *"How free do I want to be?"* It is *your* decision. And remember who else would be affected if you don't.

WHAT ABOUT YOUR DOCTOR?

DO NOT BELIEVE ANYONE, INCLUDING DOCTORS OR FRIENDS, WHO TELL YOU THAT YOU WILL HAVE TO LIVE WITH YOUR PROBLEM!

The best doctors can do is give you their *opinion* based on their *limited* knowledge. Even the best doctors don't know everything, and whatever they tell you is an educated guess based on their limited knowledge and training. This is changing slowly. Thirty-four of the 125 medical schools in the U.S.—including Harvard, Yale and John Hopkins—now offer courses in alternative medicine.

I once heard Dr. Bill McAnalley, considered by many to be the "father of glyconutritionals," share a very interesting story. During his first year of medical school, an old and wise professor made a startling announcement at the beginning of a class. He stated that one half of what they were going to learn in medical school was false—they just didn't know which half!

Don't ignore what a doctor tells you, but don't blindly believe it either. *You alone* are responsible for your health. Doctors are to be consulted by you to give you their limited perspective (opinion). Don't treat your doctor as if he or she was God.

Medical doctors have had absolutely no training on how to support the body's natural healing processes (this is slowly changing). Doctors are indeed experts and professionals in what they do, which is treating the *symptoms* of disease or trauma. *They are not trained in health or how to get it (as people often assume).*

Also, remember that the ark was built by an amateur, and the Titanic by professionals!

That your doctor knows best is a common, yet deadly assumption. You don't expect your doctor to be an expert in building houses, plumbing or fixing cars, because these are not areas in which he or she was trained. *Nor was your doctor trained in health!* Your doctor's training was in treating injuries and the symptoms of disease. Allopathic (drug based) medicine is most appropriate, and often fantastic, for accidents and a crisis situation, but it is seldom effective for treating chronic disease or restoring good health.

One example is the treatment of heart disease. Dr. Julian Whitaker states that there is no, *repeat, NO* scientific justification for the use of angiography, balloon angioplasty and bypass surgery to treat most cardiovascular disease. Several studies over the past two decades, involving over 6000 patients with heart disease, have shown that patients funneled into surgical procedures do significantly *worse* than those treated with noninvasive techniques.

A recent study on the subject was in the June 18, 1998 issue of the New England Journal of Medicine, and involved almost 1000 patients from across the country who had experienced the most common type of heart attack. Half the patients were randomly selected for invasive surgery, which included angiography and subsequent balloon angioplasty or bypass surgery. The other half were assigned to conservative management with noninvasive testing and medication. The result of this study was the same. Patients who underwent surgery did worse! The in-hospital death for heart attacks were 214% higher in the surgical group. The results of these tests are clear: *The aggressive, surgical approach does more harm than good.*

Then why do physicians keep scaring patients into these unnecessary procedures? Richard A. Lange, M.D., and L. David Hillis, M.D., suggested several factors that may be responsible, **including the financial incentives in the industry.** It may all go back to a prophesy made by Eugene Braunwald, M.D., chief of cardiology at Harvard Medical School, in 1977. Back then only 70,000 bypass surgeries were performed annually, compared to the millions of bypasses and angioplasties today.

Commenting on one of the earliest studies *that showed no benefit from bypass surgery,* Dr. Braunwald prophetically wrote, "*An even more insidious problem is that what might be considered an 'industry' is being built around this operation——-this rapidly growing enterprise is developing a momentum of its own, and as time passes, it will be progressively more difficult and costly to curtail….*"

According to the American Heart Association statistics in 1995, doctors performed 1,460,000 angiograms (the diagnostic procedure that starts the ball rolling) at an average cost of $10,880 per procedure. This resulted in 573,000 bypass surgeries at $44,820 a shot, and 419,000 angioplasties (the balloon procedure for opening up arteries) at $20,370 each. The total bill for these procedures is over $50 billion a year.

Dr. Whitaker states that much safer, noninvasive means are available for testing, monitoring, and reversing the most common forms of heart disease.

So how do you achieve vibrant health, happiness and longevity? How do you prevent or reverse disease? Is there a magic pill? Is it exercising hours every day? Is it health food? Is it positive thinking? Meditation?

Miracle Stories

Jackie Johnston ~ Fibromyalgia and Manic Depression
Over eighteen years ago I was diagnosed with fibromyalgia and manic depression. I spent two weeks at General Hospital for the depression, then a couple of years later I entered Chedoke Hospital in Hamilton, Ontario for the fibromyalgia. I stayed at Chedoke for three weeks to learn how to cope with the pain. It was a difficult task to learn because the pain was beginning to take over my brain. The doctors said I had a chemical imbalance.

I did fine for awhile, then the depression took over again. Every day when I awoke I wished I were dead. I prayed to God to help me get through the day.

I also spent three months in therapy at another rehab hospital. I thought I was getting better, but then the pain became worse than ever. I saw a counselor every week and a psychiatrist every two weeks. I was put on a lot of medication like Prozac, Amitripaline, and many others. It cost me around two to three hundred dollars each month — for medication that gave me numerous bad side effects.

My depression was getting so bad that my counselor from the rehab hospital wanted me to return to the hospital. It was around my fortieth wedding anniversary and Cheryle, my sister from Calgary, came to visit me as a surprise. She told me about one of the five strategies to vibrant health and longevity. I forgot about what she said. After Cheryle returned to Calgary, my depression got so bad I

*wouldn't get out of bed for fear I would do something bad to myself.
I just kept praying that God would take me. I didn't want to live like
that anymore.*

*I finally got desperate and called my sister. I asked her about some
of the strategies for health she had told me about. Within three days of
using one of those strategies, the fog lifted and I was no longer
depressed. I haven't suffered from depression for two years now. The
pain took awhile to go away, but my friend Margie was always there
to help me and to encourage me not to give up.*

*I now have my life back. My doctor can't believe I'm no longer
depressed. I don't see counselors or psychiatrists anymore. My husband, who now follows some of the same strategies I do, no longer has
angina attacks.*

*I've met so many wonderful people in this business of sharing the
keys to health. I am so thankful to have my life back — and I love
helping other people feel the same.*

***Shellie Todd ~ Multiple Auto-immune Diseases, Connective
Tissue Diseases, Neuro-musculoskeletal Diseases, Scleroderma,
Sjogrens Syndrome, Chronic Fatigue Syndrome, Osteoporosis,
Fibromyalgia, Diabetes, Granulomous Liver Disease,
Interstitial Lung Disease, Congestive Heart Failure, Shingles
(herpes zoster III), Vasculitis (blood vessels & veins break-
down), Chronic Arachnoiditis (sciatic nerve damage)***
*In the last three plus years, since I started using some of the strategies
to vibrant health and longevity, my life has changed in many ways!*

*By the time I started using some of the information in this book, I
was closer to death than life even though I am only forty-seven. When
Dr. Allison told me about some of the strategies for better health, I
didn't know if it was too late. I was suffering from continuous reflux
vomiting that had damaged my esophagus, making it almost
impossible for me to swallow food.*

*I decided, however, that I wasn't going to die without giving it my
best. After the first week I started feeling some major changes in my
health. But the big question was, did I make them in time? My lungs
and heart were so badly injured it was going to be a race. The doctors*

said that there was nothing they could give me to slow down the process. I was only going to live about two weeks longer.

Each time I went back to the doctors for more tests, they couldn't figure out why I was still alive — and improving to boot! Last July, when I saw my doctor for a yearly checkup, he was even more amazed than the year before. He couldn't believe I was walking and that I had driven myself the sixty miles to his office.

Life is good again! I don't want anyone to suffer any longer than they already have. I know what it's like to have lost all control over your life and health. I now have control back, and it is priceless!

My life was filled with these diseases for over twenty years. Each one was awful by itself, and when you put them all together, it was a living nightmare.

After I started to notice improvements in my health, at the end of the first week, I told my family that if I didn't make it, it was because I hadn't made the changes soon enough. I wanted them to promise that this wouldn't happen to anyone else. They had to promise me that they'd do that in memory of me!

I now have my life back and I have chosen to devote my life to seeing that others find the answers that saved my life — before it is too late for them.

When I started using some of the strategies to vibrant health I was nearly blind in my right eye and my left eye was also falling apart. It was only a matter of time before it would have to be removed. I was also in a wheelchair. I hadn't walked for two-and-a-half years.

I had high blood pressure of the lungs, which was causing congestive heart failure. But my health problems didn't end there!

I was so swollen with fluids that I was taking massive doses of water pills. But they didn't seem to help at all. I was also going into convulsions and had very slurred speech when I could talk.

My digestive system was also affected. I could hardly eat. And, what I did eat either stayed in for days or came right back up.

My liver was so large it hurt all the time. I was on a liver transplant list, but with all my other health issues, they didn't figure I'd be around to get one.

I had sixteen surgeries to try to correct some of the damage caused by my many diseases. But they were short-lived improvements. Most

*the time the surgeries caused more problems — and the need for addi-
tional surgery!*

*I can't begin to count the number of times I have been in the hospital
— nor the thousands upon thousands of dollars it has cost me, even
with health insurance. I will never be who I was before I got sick. The
years of sickness have changed me. But getting my health back using
some of the principles of vibrant health has caused even bigger
changes in me! I will never take anything for granted again.
Especially my health!*

*I have only one body, and it is mine alone to care for. For what
happens to it, happens to me. (I will feed it what it needs at any cost!
For the price of not is TOO HIGH!)*

Denise Creighton ~ Osteoarthritis

*The health recovery I've experienced has made me quite famous here
in Australia. Four years ago I was diagnosed with Osteoarthritis.
I am fifty-three years old and am an extremely active mother and
grandmother. Until two weeks ago I was a sales supervisor in an
Italian shoe boutique. I am now spreading the news full time.*

*By July 1998 I was having trouble managing the pain. Pain at rest
and range of movement was especially affected. I was getting referred
pain in the groin, and often I would just drop to the ground. I could
not kneel, and if I did, I could not get up without assistance. By the
end of the day I would be limping. My specialist told me that I was
double hip and knee replacement qualified, but because I was still so
active and the life of the new hips and knees is only ten to fifteen years,
I would just have to manage the pain and the debilitating condition.*

*Armed with a prescription for Naprosen and painkillers I left his
office. I cried all the way home. Then, in August, dosed up on my
medication, I fell off the ladder at the shoe boutique. I fractured my
sacrum and the scafoid in my left wrist. Needless to say, I was an
absolute mess. And, to add insult to injury, I was menopausal and
on HRT.*

*A friend told me about some of the strategies for vibrant health and
I decided to try them. Within four days I noticed that my arthritis pain
was less severe. It was more like a dull toothache. The pain at rest was*

significantly less and I hadn't had a groin attack. By day ten both the arthritis pain and the fracture pain were subsiding and my mobility was greatly improved. Concurrent to that, the daily hot flashes were gone and my night sweats were greatly reduced.

By the thirteenth day I was pretty much pain free — day and night. I was sitting and standing better and had more mobility around the fracture. By the end of the first month my range of movement was so improved that my five-year-old grandson Bradley commented, "Ninny, aren't you a grandma anymore?"

By the end of the second month I was totally pain free and my range of movement greatly improved. I can now run, skip, and sit on the floor with my legs crossed — things I have not done in years. I can also kneel and get up again, quickly and unaided. My menopause symptoms have totally disappeared and I am off all drugs.

It is quite obvious to me and family and friends that once properly supported, my body healed itself.

As for my son, James, he was diagnosed with Industrial Bronchiecstasis after spending six months as an apprentice spray painter using two-pack paint — WITHOUT an industrial mask. When he was eighteen we almost lost him to pneumonia and he has battled the Bronchiecstasis for six years. His medical prognosis was not good. We were told he would have continuing bouts of colds, flu, and pneumonia — and would get emphysema.

His cough and continual regime of antibiotics took their toll and he was never well. He lost weight. His skin was pale and his eyes were dull. He couldn't work and was on sickness benefit. When I introduced him to some of the strategies for vibrant health at first he balked and did not want to try them. Anyway, I insisted he give them a try.

Within four days he had a toxic cleanse. What he coughed up was unbelievable. I know because I saw the putrid, rotten, phlegm - dark brown in color and quite hard in texture. I think some of it must have been inside him for years. He consequently got a fright and told me, "Mum, you're trying to kill me," and took off. I too was concerned and called Dr. Boyd.

Dr. Boyd said, "Good, good. That means it's working."

James disappeared for four days. When I finally found him he started again. One week after that, he came into the kitchen, picked me

*up, twirled me around, and said, "THANKS, MUMMA." It was the
most wonderful moment!*

*He continues to make progress — in fact, he hardly coughs at all, he
has put on weight, he is bright-eyed and his skin is taut and has a good
color. He is working again and now has a life ahead of him. THANK
YOU, THANK YOU, THANK YOU!*

Peggy Ann Kralik ~ Arthritis, and Fibroid Tumors

*Within about two weeks of beginning to use some of the strategies to
health and longevity that a friend shared with me, my stomach problems — acid indigestion and reflux — cleared up. I haven't taken an
antacid since. And I can eat foods that I wasn't able to eat before.*

*The arthritis in my hands also cleared up. But the most remarkable
thing that happened is within four months of making some changes, my
fibroid tumors were gone! (My gynecologist verified this.)*

*Because I was so impacted by my health recovery experience, I gave
up my twenty-six-year career as a real estate appraiser and writer of
continuing education materials for appraisers in order to help people
in the way I was helped.*

Alexandra Hart-Kinney~ Osteo-arthritis

*I am forty-three and have been a teacher for nineteen years. I have
always been health conscious and tried to keep fit by exercising. But
two years ago I was told by my doctor to stop playing tennis as it was
aggravating the pain in my hips. An X-ray showed I have osteoarthritis in my hips.*

*When I asked what I could take to help my situation, several doc-
tors told me to take anti-inflammatories. One doctor was honest
enough to tell me that, although I couldn't die from the pain of osteoarthritis, I could, however, die from the overuse of anti-inflammatories. That settled it for me. I would do some research and find a
friendlier way of dealing with my situation.*

*At that time, I was also very low on energy — probably due to the
low iron level in my blood. (I had just had a complete physical exam
and discovered that I was borderline anemic.) In addition, I found*

that if I sat for longer than five minutes, my joints would almost seize up when I tried to stand.

Shortly after my arthritis was diagnosed, I ran into an acquaintance that was most excited to tell me about some strategies for vibrant health she had been using. I decided to try what she recommended.

One month later, the chronic pain in my hip joints was almost completely gone. I no longer felt stiff after sitting for a long time and I didn't have to drag myself up the stairs like an old lady any more. I could run up the stairs again! Two months later I decided to have my blood tested and was pleased to see that my iron level had returned to normal.

I had three other great "side-effects" from using some of the principles of vibrant health and longevity. Over the course of three months I found that I no longer craved sweets and gradually lost the ten pounds I had been trying to lose for five years. Also, cold sores had been a common occurrence with me — about one every four months. Since I've been on the optimal health plan I haven't had one cold sore. Who says you can't get rid of a virus?

In addition, the excruciating pains that I used to get in my legs a couple of days before a major rainstorm have virtually disappeared. This is a condition that was mild when I was a little girl, had become very severe about two years ago, and has now been eliminated. In fact, our six-year-old daughter used to regularly wake up in the middle of the night crying from the pain in her knees and would also have achy legs before a rainstorm. She started doing some of the same things I did. Now she does not have sore legs nor does she wake up in the night with aching knees. And she is certainly growing! It seemed like she was going to be the shortest in the family, but she has grown significantly in height the past two years!

Incidentally, I am playing tennis throughout the summer and am back at the level I played at twenty years ago!

James B. House ~ Advanced Metastastic Prostate Cancer
In November of 1997 I was diagnosed with advanced prostate cancer that was inoperable and that had metastasized to most of the major bones of my body - skull, spine, shoulders, upper arms, upper legs,

pelvis, and others. A bone scan showed widespread disease.

I was placed on hormone therapy - a Luprone shot every three months and flutamide pills daily. This treatment effectively killed all the male hormone cells in me, and with their destruction, all the hormone-dependent cancer cells. However, this treatment did nothing to stop the hormone-resistant prostate cancer cells which began to proliferate.

I tried the strategies for vibrant health in November of 1997 at the same time that my treatment began. A follow-up bone scan taken in May of 1999 showed a dramatic reduction in the presence of metastatic bone disease with concentrations of cancer cells in only a few localized areas. During the whole period of eighteen months I was holding down two jobs and feeling healthy. Crutches and canes are a thing of the long-ago past and I'm down to one Vicodin per day for the pain, and that just to help me sleep through it.

Sherri Louise ~ Degenerative Arthritis

In July 1994 a physician diagnosed me with degenerative arthritis. I immediately sought a second opinion. The second opinion merely echoed the first to the letter.

My symptoms included: severely swollen and red knuckles on both hands; both thumbs and forefingers beginning to turn (deform); pain from my hips (sciatica) to my knees (it felt like someone was holding a blowtorch to those areas twenty-four hours a day); and pain in my hands, wrists, forearms, and feet (so severe I no longer could interact with either of my children). All of these symptoms kept me in bed from the moment I returned home from work and every weekend.

I went to my doctors to get some relief and to find out what was going on in my body. My diagnosis was degenerative arthritis with symptomatic rheumatoid, plus carpal tunnel in both wrists, and something similar in both feet. Both doctors told me that I would need to go on prescription drugs for either the rest of my life or until my condition went into remission.

Being an ex-athlete (I was on a corporate tennis and fencing team while in my early twenties), I refused to take the drugs. My doctor advised me to get used to the pain, as there was nothing they could do for it. He did suggest that I at least go into physical therapy, at first five days a week and then to be reduced as improvement was noticed.

In late January 1995 a friend introduced me to some of the key principles of vibrant health and longevity. I asked if I could speak with someone who knew what PAIN was all about and who had also experienced relief. Three weeks later I was introduced to a gentleman from Davie, Florida, whose condition was originally actually worse than mine. He had experienced great relief from his pain.

The rest is history. Ten days after beginning with some of the strategies for vibrant health and eliminating all "night-shade" veggies, milk products and meat, and paying close attention to feeding my body appropriately, I was completely pain-free. And at four and a half months I was symptom-free! At six and a half months I was back hitting the tennis ball and at seven months I was able to get a bone density test. The test showed that my bone density was ten points higher than a healthy thirty-three-year-old woman — and at the time I was only one month shy of my fifty-third birthday.

I did go back to my original doctor to show my improvement and his comment was, "There must have been some mistake in my diagnosis!"

Never mind the fact that I no longer had any physical symptoms or PAIN! I have many times expressed my gratitude to both Susan Havener and Carol & Don Kwek for persevering in getting me the information I didn't know I needed!

2

YOUR ONLY HOPE

Your Immune System

Miracle Stories

YOUR IMMUNE SYSTEM

What do these symptoms have in common? Sore throats, runny nose, tiredness, lack of mental alertness, dizziness, unexplained weight gain, poor memory, aches and pains, low sex drive, scattered concentration, headaches, and depression. These symptoms and many more can all be associated with a poor immune function.

What do all these diseases have in common? Cancer, diabetes, asthma, atherosclerotic heart disease, auto immune disorders like lupus, hepatitis, chronic fatigue syndrome, AIDS, multiple sclerosis, osteoarthritis, fibromyalgia, Alzheimer's, and, genetic diseases like cystic fibrosis.

According to Dr. Steve Nugent, the past president of the American Naturopathic Medical Association and current president of the International Association of Complementary Medicine, the answer is:

- **They are all associated with immune system dysfunction.**
- **There is no truly effective treatment for any of these disorders.**
- **They are reaching epidemic proportions worldwide.**

The ONLY way to enjoy vibrant health, happiness and longevity is by having a strong immune system in concert with sufficient antioxidant activity. When you take care of your immune system on a holistic basis, the other critical systems will be healthy and balanced as well, including anti-oxidation, endocrine (hormonal) function, proper neurotransmitter function, and tissue repair and regeneration.

By taking care of your immune system, you can have vibrant health and longevity, and you can recover from virtually any disease. However, recovery is not possible 100 percent of the time—there is a point of deterioration (of no return).

If you were to look at a list of one hundred diseases, including heart disease, stroke, cancer, diabetes, M.S., chronic fatigue syndrome, arthritis, allergies, etc., probably over 95 percent of them will have this in common: a dysfunctional immune system.

Dr. Julian Whitaker's Perspective

Here's what one well-known medical doctor, Dr. Julian Whitaker, wrote about the immune system.

> *"For your entire life, no matter how long you may live, your body is protected by one of God's greatest miracles — your immune system. It is nothing less than your Master Strategy to All Good Health and Longevity. It consists of billions of the bravest, fiercest, most loyal centurions any emperor could ever want defending his life. These cells will literally die to protect you against any barbarian invader that threatens you.*
>
> *"Did you know that you are attacked by cancer cells every day? That's right — even if you eat nothing but the healthiest foods from pristine organic farms, the very process of digesting your food produces chemical byproducts called "free radicals." Your other metabolic functions do the same. These free radicals attack the healthy cells in your body and alter their DNA, forming cancerous cells. Allowed to replicate, any one of these cancerous cells will grow into a tumor inside you. So, every day of your life your own metabolic process produces cancer cells, which then try to set up shop and start multiplying within your body.*
>
> *Why, then, haven't you died of cancer already? Because when your immune system is strong, your loyal defender cells quickly seek out these unwanted invaders, draw their swords, engage them in battle and slay them on the spot. It happens every day of your life without any conscious effort on your part. But here's the catch...just like any other army, your internal healing army [i.e., your immune system] 'travels on its stom-*

ach.' It must have certain nutrients to maintain its fighting strength.

"And that's where we fall down. Most of us go our whole lives blissfully ignoring our brave defender 'soldiers.' It's as if we're the generals sitting on our fannies back at the officers' club far from the front. Our troops are engaged in a life-and-death struggle, sending us urgent dispatches for reinforcements and ammunition.

"But we ignore their cries for help. And sooner or later, our loyal defender cells become outgunned, overburdened, forced to defend us on too many fronts. When that happens, the tide of battle shifts...the enemies of your health gain a beachhead inside you, from which they successfully attack again and again."

Dr. Robert Adkins's Perspective

Here's a similar perspective by another medical doctor, Dr. Robert Adkins, with a particular focus on cancer as an example of what happens when you have a weak immune system.

"We've found that if you build your immune system and give it everything it needs to battle cancer, you can win the battle!

"Cancer has reached epidemic proportions, especially among people over 50. Every 45 seconds, someone dies of cancer in our country — over 500,000 per year. At this rate, cancer will be the #1 cause of death, surpassing heart disease, in less than 5 years.

"This is so shocking because 100 years ago, only one out of every 33 people ever got cancer. Today, one in three will succumb. We are heading towards one in two. Truth be told, we're losing ground. Over the last several decades, breast and colon cancer have shot up 60 percent...prostate up 100 percent...testicular up 300 percent. Even lung cancer has risen by 262 percent, at

the very time when the number of smokers has been dropping from 50 percent to 25 percent of the population.

"All this wouldn't be so terrifying if conventional medicine could deal with cancer effectively. If it could, you wouldn't fear cancer any more than you do pneumonia. But we fear cancer so much because we know, deep in our gut, that the medical establishment is powerless to help us.

"Indeed, the five-year survival rate for people who've received conventional cancer treatments has remained the same since 1950. But you have every reason for hope and optimism once you understand the real reason the medical establishment is not making progress against this disease.

"It's because for nearly 50 years, our weapons have remained the same: surgery, a variety of cellular poisonings called "chemotherapy," plus a host of techniques for blasting the body with toxic radiation. Never before in the history of medicine have such toxic "therapies" been so widely-used with such futility.

"These treatments have been pitifully ineffective for one simple reason: they assume the body's own immune system cannot be galvanized to heal itself. The assumption in the medical establishment for the past 100 years has been that cancer must be purged from the body by outside means — surgery, chemo or radiation ("cut, poison or burn").

"But chemo and radiation can wipe out your greatest hope of recovery — your immune system. This approach is an abject failure. It's time we went back to the drawing board. I, and many other MD's, now believe in battling cancer the same way we battle heart disease, arthritis, high blood pressure and other maladies. That is, by harnessing your immune system's awesome healing power, not destroying it!

"Time and again, with patient after patient, we've

found that if you build your immune system and give it everything it needs to battle cancer, you can win the battle! There are no guarantees, of course. Cancer is a powerful foe. But you can dramatically raise your odds of winning."

So how do you get a strong and healthy immune system? That's where the five strategies come in. They are your only hope to health and longevity!

Miracle Stories

Kristi Gunn ~ Daughter with Asthma

My daughter Kendie suffered from respiratory problems ever since she was born. She would throw up three to four times every night because she would cough so hard. She was diagnosed with asthma when she was a year and a half.

Kendie was put on a nebulizer, steroids, and prescription cough medicines with codeine to help control the coughing. We were very concerned about her taking all of this "poison."

My dear cousin introduced us to some of the principles of vibrant health and longevity — which we immediately began using with Kendie. Within weeks we got rid of the nebulizer, steroids, and cough medicines.

Now we all sleep every night and Kendie is as healthy as they come. We will be celebrating her second birthday next month — asthma free.

Hildegard Peschel ~ Osteoporosis, Allergies, Arthritis

I am eighty years old. In 1994 I coughed every night for four or five hours. When I breathed deeply I started to cough, so I got into the habit of doing shallow breathing. My hormone (DHEA) level was extremely low. I had osteoporosis, candidiasis, sinusitis, cataracts, allergies, arthritis, and disk trouble and angina pain. I had difficulty walking uphill because of my cough.

I experienced all of these symptoms despite living a healthy lifestyle.

I grew my own vegetables, fruits, greens, grasses, and sprouts. I juiced and ate only whole foods. After adding some of the principles of vibrant health and longevity that a friend taught me, I now feel great and am able to handle most health challenges with ease, as well as other everyday emergencies.

When my cough disappeared I practiced deep breathing. Now I can even run uphill. My DHEA level has doubled. When I drive I can see better without glasses than with. I have not been retested for osteoporosis and bone density, nor had my hearing and eyesight checked for several years. I don't see any need for it, since I am doing fine.

Jim Meyers ~ Crohn's Disease

I've been fighting Crohn's since 1988. (I am known as George Steele of the World Wrestling Federation.) It took me nine years to pin Crohn's.

My mission in life is to fight Crohn's. I talk to people all over the U.S. about my fight with Crohn's. In 1988 I was informed that I had Crohn's and that there was no cure. The disease could attack anywhere on the body from the anus to the lips. My doctor told me that my colon was destroyed and it should be removed.

This was not an option I was willing to accept. My war within was on. This was the start of my living hell. I was on as high as 120 milligrams of prednisone, Flagyl, six mp, dipentum, and Imuran. I took "moon face" to a new level.

Some of the side effects I had were drug-induced diabetes, irregular heartbeat, blood clots, cataracts, and dehydration — which resulted in a 911 call.

In 1994 I had a total bowel blockage. My colon was disconnected. I now have an ileostomy. This was not the end of my problems. After surgery I had major skin problems. I developed a hernia. I had a bout with shingles and the blood clots continued.

I have pictures of my colon from 1996 - - and it was ugly. In 1997 my doctor told me the colon had to be removed. It had gotten uglier.

Fortunately Bill Watts, a long-time friend, convinced me to try some new strategies for vibrant health. I was extremely skeptical. Bill was persistent and I tried them. After three weeks my health improved dramatically. I have my life back and even get in the ring occasionally.

In 1998 my doctor told me that I was cured and my colon could be reconnected. This was only after nine months. That gave me my life back and it is why I'm on this mission to share with others what has so changed my life.

The surgeon told me that every place I had growths, fistula and polyps, was a potential malignancy. Therefore, he said my colon should be removed. I responded that my immune system was now boosted and that my immune system would protect me from any possible malignancy. The doctor told me that because of the scar tissue my colon would never function and therefore it should be removed. I believe that my miracle is not finished yet.

Jackie Mulvey ~ Hepatitis, Pancreatitis

My senses were reeling. I had asked what was the worst and best I could hope for. The doctor said, "At worst, you could need a liver transplant in two years. At best, you might live to die of other causes."

I felt as though I had just been handed a death sentence. "Is this really happening?" I thought in disbelief. I had taught school for about twenty-four years. In 1991 I decided that I could get rich selling real estate. In fact, the trainers said that I showed the most promise of anyone in their program. Unfortunately my health didn't cooperate.

In 1992 I nearly died from misdiagnosed gallbladder problems. My health was so deteriorated by October that by the time I had surgery, what should have been simple turned into a major event. The doctors agreed there was a possibility I had pancreatic cancer.

I had been hospitalized twice with pancreatitis. I swelled so much that I appeared to be about seven months pregnant. My gallbladder had more than doubled in size and it had so inflamed everything in its vicinity that the surgery included laparotomy, cholecystectomy, trans-dudodenal sphincteroplasty, santoriniplasty, and a pancreatogram. I believe this had a dramatic influence on my immunity.

When the tubes were removed from my throat my vocal chords were so damaged I had to have speech therapy. For six months I could only whisper.

Our church had a blood drive in March 1994, and I wanted to do my part. I was in shock when the letter from the blood bank arrived stating that they would not be able to use my blood because I had non-A, non-B hepatitis. They suggested that I see my doctor.

I wondered where or when I had contracted this "death sentence." They guess that I picked up the hepatitis with blood products given to me when I nearly bled to death after the birth of my second child in 1963. (I had never been a drug user, and in 1963 blood was not screened for hepatitis.)

As I learned, anyone who received blood before 1992, IV drug users, hemodialysis patients, people with tattoos, and possibly multiple sexual partners are at risk. Body piercing and cocaine snorting are also risk factors for hepatitis C. Using razors, needles, toothbrushes, nail files, or even a barber's scissors used by infected people can transmit hepatitis.

For several months my internist kept check on my liver enzymes, which were rapidly climbing. When they went over 300, she referred me to a gastroentologist who checked the quantitative PCR RNA of hepatitis C, and did a liver biopsy. My PCR RNA was over five million, which is considered high. (This number indicates how active the virus is.) The biopsy showed that I had mild chronic active hepatitis C with some fibrosis of the liver. My enzymes climbed to around 375. That number indicated that damage was occurring.

The doctor prescribed three mil interferon three times a week. I gave myself shots in the fatty tissue of the abdomen. I experienced flu-like symptoms: headache, fever, fatigue, loss of appetite, nausea, depression, and dryness of mucus membranes. A month later, when tests indicated that I had not responded to the medication, he increased the dosage to five mil for the remainder of a twelve-month treatment. I still did not improve.

During this time all I wanted to do was go to bed and pray that I not wake up. I even thought of committing suicide. My faith in God and being afraid that I would botch the job is what prevented me from actually killing myself.

I had always been active: swimming, hiking, bicycling, etc. Now it was a struggle to climb the stairs in our two-story home. I thought my husband would need to install a lift for me to ride up and down. I didn't feel like doing anything. I didn't want to go anywhere or to see anyone. Because of the misunderstandings and lack of knowledge about hepatitis, I didn't want anyone to know I had it. I was afraid that people would think I couldn't work and would be afraid that they could catch it from me.

One of the worse parts was the isolation I felt. There was no one to talk with. I literally had to go to the library to find out about the disease.

Needless to say, my real estate career plummeted during this time. We experienced financial problems because the real estate expenses continued with little or no income.

Thank God, I heard about some principles for vibrant health through a friend, J.C. Spencer. I didn't tell him or anyone else about my health problems, but I began doing what he recommended. Almost immediately, I began to feel better.

At the end of a year, my enzymes were as low as thirteen. They have stayed normal or only slightly elevated since that time. My PCR RNA has dropped from over five mil to under one mil and is continuing to drop. The quality of my life has changed 180 degrees. I feel incredible.

I have more energy than I've had in years, and I've been able to resume all of my normal activities. I teach high school science for freshmen. I feel that God has given my life back to me through these strategies for vibrant health. I am passionate about wanting other people to know that they can have a better quality of life, too. It's great to feel good and want to live again.

Richard R. Herring ~ Allergies, Arthritis, Tuberculosis

In 1996 I was in poor health. I was on experimental drugs from the University of California Davis. I had horrible allergies and arthritis. Two years prior to that I was seen by various doctors trying to find out what was wrong with me. I was tired all the time. I had headaches and I would get nauseated. My whole body hurt, from head to toe. Even my skin hurt when I was touched.

Eventually I was diagnosed with tuberculosis. Several tests were done. The TB was in my liver. Sometimes I would crawl to the bathroom or to bed — and that's when my wife would demand to take me back to the hospital. The doctors would change my medications but I would continue to get sick. Finally I was taken off all medication and *sent home. I thought I was DYING!*

A friend came over and shared some keys to vibrant health with my wife and me. I thought it might help my wife. But, I tried it too. On the second day my allergies were gone and my arthritis was a lot better.

One day at church a friend asked me how I was doing. I told him I was doing great. My allergies were gone and my arthritis was much better. He said, "Don't you have TB or something?"

I started to cry because I realized that all of my symptoms were gone and I hadn't been to a doctor in a long time.

Since then I have had two blood tests — both were negative. I also had a lumbar puncture done, at the request of my doctor. Also a skin test. THEY WERE ALL NEGATIVE. I returned to UC DAVIS Hospital after I found out that the TB was gone. I expected that they would tell all their patients about what had worked so well for me — but I was wrong. They could care less.

THANK YOU FOR GETTING MY LIFE BACK. I didn't think I would live to see my own kids grow up. Now I am watching my grandkids grow up.

Marilyn Suni ~ Pesticide Poisoning

In September 1996, I woke up at 3 A.M. with the lower half of my body completely numb, especially the bottoms of my feet. I went back to sleep after a while and woke up at 7 A.M. I was fine. I could have sworn it was a real experience, but then I decided it must have been a bad dream.

The next night, again, I woke up at exactly 3 A.M. I had the same exact feelings of numbness in my legs, but especially at the bottoms of my feet. When I got out of bed it felt like I was walking on pointed rocks and razor blades. I stayed up for an hour and knew it wasn't a dream. I thought there must be something going on with my hormonal system and my nervous system — as if they were tied in a knot — since it happened at exactly 3 A.M. two nights in a row. I went back to sleep.

When I woke up the next morning, I was still in the same condition. It stayed that way, and I was baffled. I took good care of myself, exercised frequently, and thought I was doing all of the right things, for the most part. I had many health certifications and had done much home study in natural health over the past twenty years.

I reread all of my books, including the ones from my naturopathic course. I took many trips to the health food store to find something that would help, as if I had a cold in my nervous system, or some lightweight imbalance that would go away in a few days.

One day I had blurry vision, but not the next day. I could not feel myself urinate and things got to be quite messy when I thought I was finished, but really wasn't. My legs tingled, my liver area itched, and at times my face and forehead were numb and itched nonstop. I randomly fell and lost my balance here and there, especially when I was stressed. I ached down to my bones. (Two months before I had gone to a gynecologist because my menstrual cycles were coming two and three times per month. The gynecologist found NOTHING wrong! I was suspicious that my symptoms were a result of pesticides, as I lived in an agricultural area. I knew that pesticides mimicked estrogens, so I told the gynecologist my story...and she told me hers. I never went back again.)

I had so many weird symptoms. I can't even explain the rest of them. I waited seven days, thinking I would get better with some supplements from the health food store, but nothing changed.

I went to see a doctor. I told him that I didn't want any drugs if what I had wasn't life threatening. I told him that I thought I might have been poisoned by pesticides — either by one big blast or in small increments, as I lived in an agricultural area. The doctor said, "We only live about twenty minutes apart from each other, and if you were poisoned, I would have been poisoned, and many people would be visiting us with the same symptoms."

I was shocked. I couldn't believe he made this comment, since everyone responds differently to the same exposure, whether it is bacterial or toxic or otherwise. It also told me that doctors were not trained for general purposes in this area.

I asked for a chemical panel blood test. He said he wouldn't and couldn't do that, but I needed to see a neurologist, even though I asked for a toxicologist referral. It was very frustrating because I wasn't listened to. The neurologist did every test — except the ones I asked for. He found absolutely nothing wrong with me. I asked for a magnetic *resonance imaging of my brain, but he insisted that I have one of the spine. He found nothing wrong.*

At this point six months had passed. I researched like a mad-crazed scientist and became more and more suspicious that pesticides were poisoning me. I found threads of information but none that specifically led me to my answers. Of course, every doctor and researcher in a thousand-mile radius argued with me.

One day I finally got the chief of neurology to do an MRI of my brain, probably because he was fed up with me and wanted to shut me up. I drove about five doctors crazy with my relentless investigation. They weren't interested, but I was.

I had the MRI of my brain. That afternoon the doctor called. He was quite embarrassed when he stumbled to find the words to tell me that I had white spots in my brain and that I had suspicions of multiple sclerosis. An interesting diagnosis, using the operative word "suspicions." While I was relieved to finally get somewhere, I fell into an intense emotional state for three weeks. I was also angry because this was one of the tests I had asked for six months before.

I finally snapped out of it and continued in my quest to find out how pesticides could possibly do this destruction. I had piles and piles of articles, research reports from the University of California Davis, books, charts and labels from the agricultural products and their safety data reports on the pesticides that caused neurological and hormonal damage, and then some! In spite of everything, still the doctor said, "I am only here to diagnose and treat the symptoms."

I continued my quest, refusing to accept I had multiple sclerosis. One day I found an article that said: "MS-like symptoms caused by pesticides." With this article, I finally got the appointment I had requested for over a year, to see a toxicologist. The toxicologist actually listened to me and was suspicious that I had been right all along.

I then found out from a friend some strategies for vibrant health that I had not been aware of. I implemented them and my body's response was that all symptoms, except two, are no longer with me today.

My feet are still numb. I believe this is because some spots where the myelin used to be is not protecting my nerves. (Myelin is a fatty tissue that wraps around the nerve sheaths.) BUT, my foot bottoms are not as heavy, nor does it feel like walking on rocks and razor blades any-

more. *I have hope my feet will be normal again someday.*

My vision is also a bit blurry, but not every day. I believe this has something to do with where the myelin is missing in my brain, but I am not sure. I have all feeling back in my legs and vaginal area, normal monthly cycles, no pain, no "itchy" liver area, and no numb forehead and face.

I also used to have a difficult time speaking, remembering or find- ing words, poor memory and concentration, depression, and many other dysfunctional cognitive imbalances too weird to even describe. But no more!

When I called the chief of neurology to tell him of my recovery, he said, "Oh, it must be a coincidence!" I'll let you draw your own conclusions.

3

THE POWER OF FIRE
(The Fire Dynamic)

Your First Step

The Heart and Passion

Fulfillment & Satisfaction

Trains Need Tracks

Miracle Stories

YOUR FIRST STEP

The background against which these five strategies most effectively function is a positive and optimistic outlook on life.

According to a study reported in the American Heart Association journal, <u>Arteriosclerosis, Thrombosis and Vascular Biology</u>, middle-aged men who feel hopeless or think of themselves as failures may develop atherosclerosis, the narrowing of the arteries that leads to heart attacks and strokes, FASTER than their more optimistic counterparts.

This is *"the same magnitude of increased risk that one sees in comparing a pack-a-day smoker to a nonsmoker. Steps should be taken to try to change their situation so they gain hope or become more optimistic,"* says Susan Everson, an associate research scientist at Public Health Institute in Berkeley, California.

It is imperative that you avoid the quicksand of worry, hopelessness or even worse, pessimism. These insidious elements are like termites to your foundation. These are very large "stress checks" on your health account that lower your balance and rapidly move you closer to an "NSF" situation.

Your *foundation* for a healthy immune system and longevity is optimism. This comes from being grounded in faith, which empowers you to view life from a positive perspective, even when your circumstances are difficult (Romans 8:28). Optimism and faith are enormous deposits in your health account. It is like building your house (of health) on a solid rock instead of building it on shifting sand.

This ancient promise given by the prophet Jeremiah about 2700 years ago has brought encouragement and hope to millions of people around the world:

"I know the plans I have for you," declares the Lord, "plans for your well-being, and not for calamity, but to give you a future and a hope." Jeremiah 29:11.

THE HEART AND PASSION

The first strategy to enjoying vibrant health, happiness and longevity has to do with the heart, which is in the Fire dynamic of the 5000 year old Oriental Healing model. Three thousand years ago Solomon wrote, *"Watch over your heart with all diligence, for from it flow the springs of life."* (Proverbs 4:23).

The heart has to do with *purpose and passion.* When you have a clear compelling purpose in life you will have the fire of passion. Purpose is the only lasting source of passion. When you see yourself on a mission about which you are passionate, you will be living from your heart. You will be *"on fire."* As a result, your immune system will function far more effectively.

When you love and appreciate life and people, your natural killer cell function, which is the first line of defense of your immune system, is greatly enhanced.

Every time you feel appreciation from your heart, you are making a large deposit into your health account.

Not living from your heart, not liking your life, having no purpose and passion about anything is like having a huge IRS lien against your health account. It can be devastating. You will eventually deteriorate into a state of indifference, hopelessness and despair, and become disillusioned, cynical and bitter.

Instead of having a strong drive in the direction of your purpose, you'll be drifting aimlessly through life and end up feeling empty.

The devastating effect of this is that your immune system will be severely suppressed and compromised. As such, you are much more susceptible to virtually every health problem and disease as you start "bouncing checks."

Three thousand years ago, Solomon wrote: *"Where there is no vision (revelation), the people perish (are unrestrained); but happy is he who keeps the law."* Proverbs 29:18

Isn't it just as true today? If you don't have a clear compelling powerful revelation, that is vision of your future, you will be "unrestrained" like a car out of control about to have an accident.

The inevitable result of not having a revelation that has put you on a mission with your life is that you will "perish"—you will finish your life feeling empty, like it's all been a huge waste. Additionally, this has important spiritual application as well. And in the meantime, you will have ripped yourself off of the full potential health, happiness and fulfillment you could have had.

The second part of this ancient passage indicates that the person who follows the right principles ("the law"), such as the ones disclosed in this book, *will be happy.*

Two Life Saving Questions

One remarkable study, done by the Department of Health, discovered that the greatest predictive indicator of a fatal heart attack was not any of the traditional risk factors, such as smoking, high cholesterol or obesity. It could be most accurately determined by the answers to two simple questions: *"Are you happy with your life?"* and *"Do you love your work?"*

A startling discovery also was made in this study. The most likely day and even the time to have a heart attack was predictable. Any guesses? Most heart attacks occur on Mondays. And the time? You probably guessed it! At 9 a.m.!

What does this tell you? *That people would rather die than go to work!*

The point is, if you don't love your work and feel passionate about it, and if you are not happy with your life (because you are not making a meaningful contribution), you'd better start thinking about making a drastic change before it is too late! If you don't love what you do, find what you do love to do, and start doing it! It's never too late to start, even if you are in your eighties!

Plus, when you live as if you are on an important mission (and I believe you are), you can't afford to take time to get sick because what you are doing is so important to you.

"Dear God, what is my purpose here?"

The USA Today newspaper reported the results of a survey in which adults were asked what question they would ask God if they could get a direct and immediate answer. Over two thirds responded with a question relating to their purpose, and half of those would ask specifically, *"What is my purpose here?"*

If having passion that comes out of having a clear sense of purpose and destiny is lacking in your life, I strongly recommend that you start looking immediately for something that you can really put your heart into, some cause over which you can be on fire! Find a project or a business through which you can make a meaningful contribution AND love what you are doing. When you make a positive difference for others, by contributing to their lives in a meaningful way, not only is your value and personal worth affirmed, but you will be happier. As a result of that, your immune system will be stronger and you will be that much closer to having health, happiness and longevity.

A powerful first step in creating a purpose with passion is to identify your core values. An easy and fun way to do this is to do a short exercise created by one of my mentors, Mike Smith. Just go to www.bridgequestinc.com or request a free Web-Disk by calling (800) 449-9488. Also, consider taking the life changing "Freedom Course" by BridgeQuest. It made a very major and lasting change for me for which I will always be grateful.

The four most helpful books I've read on developing your purpose and passion are:

- Unstoppable by Cynthia Kersey
- Living With Passion – 10 Simple Secrets That Guarantee Your Success by Peter Hirsch
- The Joyful Spirit – How to Become the Happiest Person You Know by Brian Biro
- Get A Life – How to Leave That Dead-End Job Behind and Create Your Perfect Future – Today! by Philip Stills

My favorite book on developing a personal vision and self-motivation is <u>Mach II With Your Hair On Fire</u> by Richard Brooke. These powerful books can help you "catch on fire" by developing a passionate purpose in life. The best audio tapes that I have found on this subject are by John Maxwell, entitled, <u>Vision—The Process of Passing it On</u>.

My personal ultimate purpose and passion in life is to make God happy. A major part of that is to make a significant difference for millions of people by supporting them in achieving better health, happiness and fulfillment, and in supporting them to help others in the same way. I love doing this so much, I've made it my business so I can do it all the time. I don't need to work anymore for money, but I do work on my purpose.

I am a man on a *mission*. It's my passion and a major source of my happiness, satisfaction and fulfillment. That's why I've written this book. I love to educate, equip and empower others and do it in a way that they can educate, equip and empower others too.

I invite you to join me in this mission of making a significant difference for people. It is one of the most rewarding and fulfilling things you can do with your life!

FULFILLMENT & SATISFACTION

My personal belief is that every human being is driven by the desire to feel *valuable, significant and important*. This is the basic universal drive that runs us. Everyone wants to be "somebody."

Of the countless ways we try to affirm our personal value, many of which do not work well, the two that are most effective and fulfilling are *contribution* and *connectiveness*.

When we make a *contribution* to the lives of others, we are the most happy and fulfilled because this *affirms and reinforces* our own value and significance.

When we feel *connected* to others, which includes a sense of belonging and being loved, we are happy and fulfilled, because this too *affirms* our value and significance. When *contribution* and *connectiveness* encompass the spiritual realm, we are the most happy and fulfilled!

Heart Amplification

To get the most value from the other four strategies, engage your heart by doing them with a conscious focus on your *physical* heart. Whatever you do, do it with and through your heart from a sense of *appreciation*.

Years of research have shown that by simply doing this, you can raise immune function levels (as measured by the IgA (immunoglobulin A) by an average of 34 percent and increase the amount of the hormone DHEA (considered to be an anti-aging hormone) available to the cells by up to 100 percent, while decreasing the cortisol (the stress hormone) by 23 percent. I use this dynamic of appreciation every day, and it only takes me a few seconds to use it with wonderful benefits.

This stress reducing and health building technology is fully explained in the HeartMath Technology materials that are available at www.heartmath.com or by calling (800) 700-1238 or (888) 666-8942. I strongly recommend learning this simple and powerful life enriching technology for bringing purpose and passion into your life so you can be making significant deposits daily into your health account.

Another important aspect of living from your heart is to enjoy uplifting and inspirational music. In fact, music can be very healing, especially when you sing to it. Positive music is a great daily deposit in to your health account.

Laugh Your Way to Health

A final aspect of living from the heart is to smile and laugh a lot, especially with the people you care about the most. We tend to take life too seriously which is a stress check against our health account. Enjoy life. Be grateful. Look for or make up reasons to celebrate! Create excitement and adventure. Look for the humor in situations, even if you have to look really hard. Tell jokes. Be funny.

Some people "laugh" at their future, at the possibility of having a meaningful fulfilling life. This kind of laughter is based on cynicism and unbelief, and could cause you to forfeit your destiny. Instead, laugh at your doubts and the limited reasoning that says you can't have a wonderful and fulfilling life. Save your laughter for celebration and fun!

The father of laughter therapy is Norman Cousins. He had an incurable disease, ankylosing spondylitis. His pain was so high that even morphine would not help. He discovered that ten minutes of belly laughter would give him enough relief to sleep for two hours. He went on to a full cure and lived an additional twenty years pain free because he learned how to use laughter to stimulate the immune system.

When he was in the hospital with this incurable disease, he had a nurse that was assigned to him to take care of him. This particular nurse was one of these "we" people. She'd start the day by saying, "And how are we feeling today" or "We need a urine sample" etc.

Norman did not like her, so one morning when they brought his breakfast, he poured his apple juice in the urine cup. Later when the nurse came in and picked up the urine cup, she said, "My, we have cloudy urine this morning, don't we?" He said, "Give me that. I'll run it through again" and swallowed it. She quit! She refused to take care of him anymore, saying he was crazy.

Research has demonstrated that the positive effects of laughter not only decrease stress and certain neuroendocrine hormones but spontaneously increase the activity of natural killer cells that are vital to fighting and preventing disease (see <u>Humor & Health</u> November/December, 1994 issue, Volume III, Number 6).

A research study was presented at the Psycho Neuro-Immunology Research Society Meetings on April 18, 1996 in

Santa Monica, California by Stanley Tan M.D., Ph.D. and Dr. Lee Berk. The study's experimental group consisted of ten healthy, fasting adult male volunteers. They viewed a preselected sixty-minute mirthful/humor video. Blood samples for gamma interferon (IFN) were obtained through an IV catheter. IFN was measured before the subjects viewed the humor video (baseline), during (intervention), after (recovery) and also the following day.

The data revealed a significant increase in the activation of T cells, B cells and increases in immunoglobulins and natural killer cell activity. For more information on how to customize laughter to get the maximum health benefits, visit www.touchstarpro.com/wellness.html.

It is still true, that "A *joyful heart is good medicine, but a broken spirit dries up the bones.*" Proverbs 17:22

TRAINS NEED TRACKS

This first strategy, based on the Fire dynamic, has to do with purpose, passion and living from your heart. Here's an analogy to help you with some further insight into how the Fire dynamic applies to your life and health.

Picture your health as a strong and magnificent locomotive pulling a number of cars full of treasure and other valuable cargo. This train is on an important mission, perhaps even a mission from God. It has a purpose and a destiny. This train also has an important role in a larger plan.

The person driving this train is you. Because you fully understand this purpose and the valuable contribution your train can make in the larger scheme of things, you are passionate about reaching the intended destination. In fact, to use another metaphor, you are "on fire" to fulfill your mission, and are thus living from your heart.

Obviously, for things to go well, your train must be on the tracks. **These tracks represent your purpose in life.**

What do we call it when a train goes off the tracks? A train wreck!

So for you to avoid a train wreck and reach your destiny, you've got to *be* on the right track, and *stay on track!* And if you are not "on track" now with any particular destination, NOW is the time to figure it out and get back on track!

Miracle Stories

Michael A. Currieri, Ph.D. ~ Cancer

I am a psychologist. I specialize in brain functional analysis (brain mapping) and rehabilitation using biofeedback and neurofeedback, a wonderful form of alternative therapy that trains the brain to enhance performance. I also work with injury and pain patients, again using alternative treatment with an instrument called the Acuscope that uses microcurrent to heal at the cellular level.

In the summer of 1997 I began a rigorous training program to prepare for a cross-country bicycle trip. It was a fundraising event for the American Lung Association. While I have always kept myself in pretty good condition and always followed a fairly good nutritional regime, I knew I was not prepared for a 3,400-mile, six-and-a-half week bicycle event.

I planned out the next ten months carefully and began a training program that included an ever-demanding exercise and bicycling program. I joined a gym and worked with a professional trainer. I began paying more attention to my eating and increased the nutritional products I was already taking. I charted every day and tracked my progress. I felt my body getting stronger and my confidence growing.

In late May of 1997 I was ready to begin one of the biggest adventures of my life. We, over a thousand of us, were scheduled to 'launch' on June 15, starting from Seattle and ending in Washington D.C. forty-five days later. I felt strong and eager to begin. My training had steadily advanced and I could now easily hop on my bike and cover one hundred miles any time I wanted.

One week before 'launch' I noticed a lump on my neck that had been hiding under my beard. I felt a jolt of fear course through me. I pushed down the ugly thought of what this might mean. Cancer ran in my family. But no, not me. It couldn't be. It isn't. I just knew it.

I went to a doctor friend. He said it was just a swollen lymph node. "Go on your bicycle trip," he said. "Don't worry." I felt relieved. I had heard what I wanted to hear. But a nagging voice echoed deep within me. A dear friend of mine insisted I get a second opinion. I resisted. I did not want to go. She insisted. She was relentless.

The second doctor also believed it was nothing — but decided to take a biopsy just to be sure. Thus began the most terrible and frightening event of my life. A tumor was discovered on the base of my tongue. The cancer had spread to the lymph nodes on both sides of my neck. I was paralyzed with fear and denial. The nightmare had begun.

On July 7, 1998 I had surgery at the University of Washington. It was a brutal surgery and required many hours of intensive and intrusive work to remove the cancer. Even though I was in excellent physical condition, my body was devastated by the trauma of the surgery.

The following months proved to be a living hell. I couldn't swallow anything. I had to be fed through tubes. I couldn't sleep because I could not swallow the saliva and phlegm that gathered and gagged me in my throat. My weight dropped, my spirits dipped, my hope of survival and a normal life dimmed.

Six weeks after the surgery I was told I would now have to begin a series of radiation treatments. The radiation would cause permanent damage to the sensitive areas in my mouth and throat. My taste buds and salivary glands would be destroyed. I would likely loose teeth and possibly jawbone. I would forever more be subject to easy infections. I talked with people who had gone through radiation in the throat and mouth area. Some had to forever be fed with a tube because they could not swallow anything except water. All of them suffered digestion problems and continual dry mouth because of the loss of their salivary glands. They said food tasted like cardboard. I thought of the wonderful Italian dishes I loved cooking and eating. I would never taste them again.

There were other risks and losses. I heard of poor unfortunate people that had undergone the terrible surgery and radiation only to have the cancer return. I told the doctors I was unwilling to damage my body to such an extent. I would not do radiation. I would find another way. I was told in no uncertain terms, "You are a fool and will likely die a miserable, long suffering death."

Just prior to surgery my blood samples showed T, B and NK cells reactivity to be very low: T cell reactivity was one with normal expected to be twenty to twenty-nine. B cell reactivity was one with normal expected to be ten to twenty-nine. NK cell reactivity was 528. With normal expected to be above 40,000.

By now I had just about given up on medical doctors. They did not have any solutions. They frightened me by telling me of the awful death I would suffer if I did not submit to radiation treatments, that what I was doing was sub-standard care. I argued radiation would suppress my immune system even further; would damage me beyond reason, and offered no assurance of protection. "That's all there is. This is state of the art," I was informed. I was given a prescription for an antidepressant and sent home. I did not take the prescription, fearing it would shut my system down even further.

Then in late December of 1998, some dear friends of mine, Virginia and Bill Talbot, shared some new technology on how to dramatically support the immune system, which was exactly what I needed.

Cautiously, I began to feel optimism build. "Don't get your hopes up," the "Vultures" (what I call the shrill voice of fear) inside my head screamed at me. "This is all just hype. Maybe it worked for them, but it won't for you." I pushed the mistrust down. It would not stay put. Doubt surfaced at every opportunity and washed over me. Fear and uncertainty of recovery had taken deep roots and would not be so easily expelled.

I gave it a try. Approximately ten days later I sensed more than felt a slight change. My body, especially in my chest area, felt lighter and more open. The "Vultures" came out and smugly told me it was my imagination.

But I definitely felt better. My appetite was ravenous. I had not really felt hunger since the days of my 100-mile bike training trips. My body was not as cold as it had been. I could even take off the sweatshirt and gloves I often wore indoors. I felt more energetic and the terrible depression was lighter and lifted daily. The constant fear and the "Vultures" always lurking in the background were withdrawing.

On January 26, 1999, I got the test results from a blood sample taken — just twenty days after I started with the changes I had made. My T cells, B cells and NK cells were all in the normal range. The NK cells shot up from 1,027 to 51,545. The doctor from the Immunocomp Lab called me and said, "Whatever you are doing, keep doing it." I told him about what I was doing and he said, "Send me some information. I'm interested in this."

I am thrilled to share this information with my family, my loved ones, and anyone who will take the time to listen. I feel a growing delight inside. I believe I will indeed have the opportunity to complete my bicycle adventure. Only this time it will be with a stronger fully nourished body and a wiser peaceful mind, knowing I have taken responsibility for the guardianship of what God has provided me.

One last thing. When I discovered I had cancer, I was in the best physical condition of my life. I was prepared for an endurance marathon of major proportions. There was no hint of illness. If someone had told me about how to improve my immune system then, I may not have listened. I may have thought, "What need do I have for that?" I was, after all, in top condition, ready to ride my bicycle across America.

However, if someone had shared these ideas with me a few years ago, and if I would have had the wisdom to listen to them and to make some changes, two things may have happened. Likely I would not have had to deal with cancer, and likely I would be a very wealthy man today.

The thought keeps going through my head, 'When Noah built the Ark, it wasn't raining.' So now I will say to anyone who will listen, "Take care of yourself now while you still feel healthy. Don't try to play 'catch up'. It's too hard."

One more very important thing has dramatically changed for me since I started using strategies for vibrant health. I have had moderate to severe asthma since childhood. I had to use three different medication inhalers to have normal breathing. Sometimes I had to use this medication eight or nine times a day. My sleep was often disturbed because of wheezing and difficult breathing. I no longer have a breathing problem. There is no sign of shortness of breath or wheezing. I have not touched my medication since I made the changes.

I am now back in my practice working with clients, and am now beginning to train for the "Bike Across America" adventure next year. Also, I am sharing what I have learned with as many people as possible.

Debbie Jmaeff ~ Depression, Suicidal, Violent Behavior
I have suffered from depression all of my life. For as long as I can remember I felt as if people were out to get me. I was always sick and lived a miserable life going back and forth from doctors to psychologists.

Shortly after I was married I got pregnant with my son, Devon. About halfway through the pregnancy I became severely depressed, although I didn't realize it at the time. After his birth the depression turned into postpartum depression. I was withdrawn, had sudden mood swings, violent at times. I sought help but there was none - - except for people telling me to "just get over it." I did see a natur-opath, who provided some relief — although I was never totally depression free. I frequently felt like killing my son and myself.

When Devon was thirteen months old I became pregnant again. This time, since I was already depressed, I became suicidal, violent, and unpredictable much sooner, somewhere around seven and a half months into the pregnancy. Again no one said they could help.

After my daughter, Lindsey, was born I became extremely volatile. One day I was at my neighbor's house and my son did something that upset me. I flew into a rage and dragged him home while carrying my screaming two-month old. When we reached our front door I became violent with my son. Once inside the house, after considerable scream-ing and almost killing my own child, I realized something was wrong.

I called the hospital and my naturopath. My husband came home from work. I was finally diagnosed with chronic depression, severe postpartum depression. Everyone wanted to put me on Prozac but I refused. I knew that wasn't the answer and I didn't want to quit nurs-ing my daughter. I went to my naturopath for extensive testing. There it was determined that I have a neurotransmitter disorder. I was treated naturally and found great relief, although not permanent — and it was costing a small fortune!

About six months later a friend of my husband told me about one of the strategies for vibrant health and longevity. At first I wasn't sure, because I had tried everything else and nothing seemed to work for very long. But he was a good friend so I decided to try it.

Within one week I felt major changes in my body. Within three weeks

I was off one of the natural medications I was taking daily and within four weeks I was completely off everything! My naturopath was testing me through this whole process and was astounded by the results. This was the first time in my entire life that I actually felt calm, well, and normal. I had never, ever felt like this before.

Now, two years later I feel terrific and do not fear any recurrence of my previous symptoms. I am pregnant again and the doctor says I have never been so healthy and adjusted. I know I will be fine this time — thanks to these principles of health.

Don Wells ~ Wife's Pituitary Gland Tumor, PMS

My wife, Leslie was diagnosed as having a pituitary gland tumor in 1991. It was obvious from the magnetic resonance imaging that it had been affecting her for some time. This was the first time we connected the mood swings and severe premenstrual syndrome with a physical problem.

My wife struggled with the symptoms for up to two weeks a month. Three to four days during this period I would come home from work and find her in a fetal position, crying. Although we fought constantly during these periods I do not remember what we fought about! If I only understood then what I know now, I could have been much more supportive!

Other symptoms included migraines that started from the back of her head at the tip of her spine, to terrible body aches and cramps. All this from the moment she got up to when it was time for sleep — if you could call it sleep.

An artificial hormone replacement therapy (parlodel) was prescribed. The symptoms at this point took a turn for the worse and became amplified. We were told that there was no other choice, except for surgery under the nose and between the eyeballs to extract the lump.

Leslie's doctor told us that if we chose the operation, the potential long-term side effects could be dementia, diabetes and a few other "d" words that I could not understand at the time. The symptoms seemed easier to deal with than the operation, so we stuck with the drugs.

In 1996 Rick Woelinga and Dianne Vincent introduced us to some strategies for vibrant health that we had not heard of before. Leslie

*started in the spring of 1996. Three weeks later 100 percent of
her symptoms virtually disappeared. It was that dramatic. The
fourth month regressed to old habits and all the symptoms started to
reappear. On the fifth month we changed our priorities! All the
symptoms disappeared again. In September 1996 Leslie stopped
using parlodel.*

*At this same time I told my brother, Dwight, and his wife, Judith,
about the amazing results Leslie was having and that Dianne was
eager to give me information on a family who had positive results
using one of the principles of vibrant health for a person with a rare
disorder called Tourette's. Dwight and Judith's son, Everette, had
suffered tremendously with this and consequently was tearing the
family apart.*

*Within six months their son went through a metamorphosis. To
this day you could not tell him apart from any other teenage boy. It is
an amazing story unto itself. Everette was also able to get off all
prescribed drugs.*

*Both of my daughters have seen great things happen when they
began incorporating some of the strategies for vibrant health —
everything from reduced illness, infection, and asthma to greater
mental clarity.*

*In February 1999 my wife got the results back from her latest
computerized axial tomography (CAT) scan. As I suspected, the tumor
was gone. What a strange feeling overcame us. Leslie was quiet all
weekend, as I was euphorically quiet (screaming inside). It was like
a continuous release of pressure with no end in sight. We had our
future back!!*

Jim and Minta Owsley ~ Fibromyalgia
*Nine years ago my wife, Minta, was diagnosed with fibromyalgia. Her
doctor prescribed medications for Minta for three years. She almost
became addicted to them. After four and a half years, Minta's health
began to decline drastically. She was close to being bedridden.*

*In July 1998, Minta applied for Permanent Disability. At this time
our son told us about the strategies to vibrant health and longevity.
Skeptical at first, Minta said she would try them - - if I did too.*

*A month later Minta felt like something was going on inside of her.
Two weeks later she literally peeled off a layer of dead skin (toxins)
from her stomach area. This convinced us that healing had begun.*
*The rest is history. Minta works forty hours a week and walks
two to four miles every Saturday. Before, she could barely walk up
the driveway.*

Sharon Skalenda ~Rheumatoid Arthritis/Fibromyalgia

*Five years ago I began to swell in different joints. My right arm was
constantly swollen from my hand up to my elbow. The pain and stiffness gradually worsened. I literally hurt from the top of my head to the
bottom of my feet. It was painful to brush my teeth and to comb my
hair. I became so weak I couldn't lift the sheet off me in the morning.
After three months of trying every vitamin available, I made an
appointment to see a rheumatologist. The diagnosis was fibromyalgia.
He gave me a cortisone shot because my left hand was so swollen my
wedding band was cutting into my finger. I had four to six weeks
reprieve from the pain.*

*In the months that followed I pursued natural remedies. I would
endure three horrible months of pain and then be slightly better for the
next three months. This pattern continued until someone sent me information on a formula for fibromyalgia. Within twenty-four hours I
was much better, and I continued to improve for almost a year.*

*Then, in February 1998, completely out of the blue, I got sick
again. I endured three horrible months of pain and stiffness. I was
barely able to function. I kept thinking I could overcome this again - -
but nothing I took made the slightest difference. I finally went to
another rheumatologist. He said he couldn't do anything for the
fibromyalgia except prescribe muscle relaxants and/or antidepressants.
I wanted neither.*

*Later that evening he called me about the results of some blood tests
he had ordered. He wanted to see me immediately. My sed rate was
100 (normal is 0 to 20), and the other tests results were elevated too.
He started my on Prednisone and Plaquenil, with a diagnosis of
rheumatoid arthritis. He ordered a retest for lupus. Because I was in
such terrible pain I agreed to the medications - in hope of some relief.*

Within twenty-four hours my pain had lessened.

However, as the pain subsided and I was able to think more clearly, I knew I had to get off these medications. I had gained forty pounds from the Prednisone. I feared the toxicity of the meds. That night I sat at my computer and prayed to God for guidance in finding relief. Eventually I came upon some information on the strategies for vibrant health. I decided to try it.

I immediately felt an improvement in my energy level. Whenever I slacked off using the strategies, I could feel a setback in my health. I feel significantly better now - - and am only taking 2.5 milligrams of Prednisone now. I still have a ways to go - - but the last two months I have felt almost normal - - a feeling I did not imagine I would ever have again.

4

MAKING YOUR
CONNECTION
(The Earth Dynamic)

Being Well-Connected

Trains Need Connections

Miracle Stories

BEING WELL-CONNECTED

The second strategy to vibrant health, happiness and longevity is associated with the Earth dynamic. The Earth dynamic represents having a sense of *connectedness* with others.

Your immune system is stronger when you feel connected to other people in relationships where you feel valued, respected and loved. Every time you feel connected with someone, another large deposit has been created and put into your health account. Ideally, if you are married, you feel well connected with your spouse. If this is not your experience, it is worth working on as one of your more important health goals.

If you are single, or if connectedness is not achievable in your marriage, it can be achieved through a community of people who share a common vision, such as a church, organization or a business that is based on a cause or mission.

Even if you have a great marriage, you still need and can benefit greatly from being a part of a broader based community of people who love and respect you and with whom you share a common purpose and mission.

The Terrible Price for being "Disconnected"

The default and all too common alternative to being connected with people is aloneness, isolation and insecurity. These are very serious withdrawals from your health account.

Quite often what keeps people from being part of a loving community of people is a fear of not being accepted, or blame and bitterness, which can fuel self-imposed isolation.

The unavoidable consequence of *not* being connected with people is once again a compromised immune system, which will most likely keep you in that 95 percent category.

If there is a way to be *"on fire" with passion* about a cause or significant purpose (mission) and "grounded" (to the Earth) by being connected to others in a community of believers, your chances for having vibrant health and longevity will be greatly increased.

It is my personal belief, that the most important person to be connected to is God.

The opposite of connection is disconnection or *separation*, and separation is the biblical definition of death. If separation and disconnection are characteristic of *any* area in your life, you are "dead" in that area, whether it be socially, emotionally or spiritually. And if you are not well connected internally (immune system, cell to cell communication, hormones, etc.), you are most likely going to be dead physically that much sooner.

"There is overwhelming evidence that people who have few social contacts are more likely to get sick and less likely to recover from an illness," says Erik Peper, Ph.D., Associate Director of the Institute of Holistic Healing Studies at San Francisco State University.

In fact, a nine-year study reported in the Journal of Epidemiology (Feb. 1979) that people with the lowest amount of social ties were *two to three times more likely to die of all causes than those with the most social connectiveness!*

The High Price of Social Inequality

Thirty years of scientific research has established that the most powerful predictor of human disease is social and economic inequality. In the past 5 years, 193 studies have been published on various aspects of socioeconomic status and health, according to the New York Times.

As the New York Times reported June 1, 1999 in its weekly Science Section,

"Scientists have known for decades that poverty translates into higher rates of illness and mortality. But an explosion of research is demonstrating that social class — as measured not just by income but also by education and other markers of relative status — is one of the most powerful predictors of health, more powerful than genetics, exposure to carcinogens, even smoking."

A sense of opportunity, dignity, self-esteem, the respect of others — all these are important for health. Social cohesion — a sense of neighborliness — also plays a role: people live longer in places where they believe they can trust their neighbors.

As Harvard economist Juliet Schor says, *"The reasons may not turn out to be so very complicated. Humans are social. We judge our own situations very much in comparison to others around us. It is not surprising that people experience less stress, more peace of mind, and feel happier in an environment with more social cohesion and more equality."*

See Appendix section 14 for more information on this important aspect of health.

Add Eight Years to Your Life!

One study, published in the May 1999 issue of the <u>Journal Demography</u>, found that, in general, people who attend worship services one or more times each week live about 8 years longer than those who never attend religious services.

This report showed that people who never attend church live to about 75, while those who attend services one or more times a week live to an average age of 83.

The study, which analyzed data from the National Health Interview Survey, also found that those people who never attended religious services had an *87% higher risk of dying from all causes* during a 9-year follow-up period than those who attended services one or more times per week.

Evidently, taking regular time to connect with God and others in a church setting on a weekly basis creates such a major weekly deposit into your health account that it is measurable to the tune of eight extra years of longevity!

Two thousand years ago, we were given the same advice: *"Confess your faults to one another, and pray for one another, so that you may be healed"* (James 5:16) and *"...think of ways to stimulate each other to love and good deeds, not forsaking our own assembling together, as is the habit of some, but encouraging one another...."* (Hebrews 10:24-25).

TRAINS NEED CONNECTIONS

This second strategy, based on the Earth dynamic, has to do with Connectiveness. Let's build a little further on the train analogy to give you some further insight into how the Earth dynamic applies to your health.

Besides needing tracks to run on (your purpose), a train needs to be well connected to the earth through the tracks. If this vital connection is lost, the mission will be aborted. Furthermore, if your train attempts to operate in isolation from others without regular service and maintenance, it will eventually break down and grind to a halt.

Also, if your train engine loses the connection to the cars of cargo it is pulling, even if it reaches the destination, the trip will have been in vain.

Plus, a single person is not capable of operating a train. An entire crew is needed. You've got to have a well-connected team that supports you and your mission, or else the entire mission is jeopardized.

Miracle Stories

Corrie Snieder ~ Diabetes, High Blood Pressure

I had lived with diabetes for over thirty-six years and was taking insulin three times a day. I had diabetic related renal disease and eye problems, five coronary bypasses ten years ago, and a heart attack five years ago. My doctors assured me that the complications from the diabetes would only worsen, and a tear in my left rotation cuff meant that I would never regain full use of my arm. They didn't know why my knee hurt - - I'd have to live with it.

I was seriously looking for something to make me feel better. After trying various "health" foods, I tried the strategies for better health. Three months later I noticed that my sugars were going down, my blood pressure was down, and the pain in my knee had lessened.

Things just kept getting better. My insulin requirements are down 20 percent, I'm off all blood pressure medicine, and my knee is pain-free.

Also, my eyes have improved so much I need a weaker prescription. And, I now have full use of my left arm. Basically, I have a lot more energy and am enjoying life much more.

Janis Holt ~ Chronic Headaches

For four years I suffered from chronic headaches twenty-four hours a day. On a scale of one to ten, the pain averaged a seven or an eight. I visited a variety of healthcare professionals, including neurologists, chiropractors, and acupuncturists. I underwent sinus surgery and had allergy injections. I tried many herbal remedies and numerous over the counter medications. In January 1996 a doctor asked if I was interested in taking something else to treat my headaches. Of course I said yes. After a couple months I started feeling better and was able to wean myself off of the pain killers. Now, I am doing great!

Stacie Smith ~ Self and Family Members with Uncontrolled, Eating, Hernia, Chronic Depression, Fibromyalgia

In 1998 my father was very sick with fibromyalgia, chronic depression, and had the beginning signs of Alzheimer's. Friends of the family introduced my parents to the strategies for vibrant health. Within two days my father noticed an incredible difference. He could reach into his back pocket - - something he had not been able to do for years. His whole attitude was different. It was like I had gotten my father back after all these years.

Equally as amazing was my mother's transformation. I had never noticed how bad her addiction to sweets had become (she was to the point that she vomited every night because she ate so much junk). In six months she lost fifty pounds and is off Prozac for depression. She no longer takes estrogen and looks incredible!

After seeing my parents' improvements, my entire family tried the strategies. My husband had a hernia, high blood pressure, and chronic heartburn. Now the hernia is nonexistent, and he no longer takes anything for high blood pressure or heartburn.

I used to suffer from allergies so badly that I had painful sores in my nose. I was also on Prozac for chronic depression. Now, the strate-

gies have made us all better. Nothing has changed my life like this!

Pamela Desilets ~ Severe Cervical Whiplash

In October 1996 I was rear-ended while stopped at a stoplight. Within one hour after the accident I was in severe pain. I had suffered a severe cervical whiplash. Thus began my journey into insomnia. I lived in pain every day - - but at night, when I tried to sleep, it worsened. Hence, no sleep. Eventually I developed migraine headaches that would last for up to three days. Soon I had to forgo my weightlifting program, and running became difficult.

At this time my boss, a chiropractor, was treating me up to four times a week with various types of manipulations and physical therapies. I also had physical therapy with a registered physical therapist for a couple of months. And, I visited my regular doctor, who prescribed various drugs, which, in addition to producing negative side effects, did not relieve the pain.

Very reluctantly I had to quit running. Then walking became painful, and then sitting became uncomfortable. In September 1997 my bilateral arm pain was so severe I returned to the doctor. This time he diagnosed me with chronic fatigue syndrome and fibromyalgia. It was a relief to finally put a name on my ailments.

Fed up with traditional medicine, I began to search for alternative treatments. In October 1997 I read an article in a home school magazine about a woman and her success with strategies to health. I contacted her that night and asked her about the strategies.

At about six weeks I started having more energy. At nineteen months I have experienced additional health benefits: improvement in my allergies, sinus and bowel problems; softer skin; and a reduction in premenstrual syndrome symptoms. In June 1998 I competed in a 5.2-mile race. To me, that was a miracle.

Shauna O'Neill ~ Stress/Fibromyalgia/Asthma

One and a half years ago I was under a lot of stress and started to develop symptoms of fibromyalgia. I became depressed from the pain and immobile. My hair began to thin due to stress. I was very weak, shaky, and suffered from memory loss and numbness. As a nurse I believed medicine could help. However, after seeing a dozen doctors and trying every medication and test to ease my symptoms, I was no better off. I felt like I was slowly dying and losing my mind. No one understood or could help me.

I finally gave in to my girlfriend, who suggested I try principles of vibrant health . In two weeks I began to notice some relief. After three months I felt a lot better, I had more energy. After five months I noticed my asthma was better. After a year my hair started coming back. I would say I am 80 percent better. My life has truly changed forever!

Jo Lynne Wells ~ Fibromyalgia

Since about 1994 I have suffered with severe fatigue, muscle aches, headaches, insomnia, and depression. The fatigue bothered me the most because I would sometimes be so weak I could barely stand. By the summer of 1996 my symptoms were so bad I couldn't work for four months - - a very scary situation for a single mother with two boys.

My doctor said she could find nothing wrong with me, except that I was depressed. She referred me to another doctor, who prescribed anti-depressants, including lithium. When I complained to the doctor that I actually felt worse, he simply increased the dosage of the drugs. As my symptoms continued to worsen I requested that he test for some other illness. The doctor suggested electric shock therapy. After that suggestion I quit seeing the doctor and took myself off the drugs.

Of course, that didn't solve my severe fatigue. I prayed for several years that I would find an answer. I went to a rheumatologist and it was determined that I had fibromyalgia. I had tried several food sup-plements, which didn't work. So, when I met Denise Romero and she told me about the strategies for vibrant health, I was skeptical. But by the end of ninety days I was convinced that I was improving. I am so thankful!

Linda Ott ~ Allergies/Sinus Infections/Bronchitis

For over twenty years I felt rotten. I continually had allergies, sinus infections, bronchitis, ulcers, anemia, fatigue, aches and pains, and

*depression. Many doctors in six different states tried to find out
what the cause of these problems were. They all said the same thing - -
depression.*

*In September 1997 a new family physician diagnosed fibromyalgia
and suggested I try the strategies for vibrant health. After trying the
strategies for three months I realized I was not taking a nap every
day. And I hadn't been to a doctor for a sinus infection or bronchitis
in months. By the end of a year I no longer needed the two allergy
medications, the medication for ulcers, or the medication for depression. And, I had no more food cravings! My body fat dropped from
27 percent to 19 percent! I had a life once again.*

Jerry Tufte ~ Arthritis

*Several years ago my knee was injured playing basketball. An orthope-
dic surgeon told me I had the knee of an eighty-year-old. I was thirty-
eight at the time. I was too young for knee replacement surgery, so I
just had to live with the pain.*

*My wife, Donna, had been in an automobile accident, so she too
was facing many physical problems.*

*A close friend of ours suggested the principles of vibrant health for
both of us. After only two weeks the pain in my knee was gone - - even
after standing on it all day. Donna experienced tremendous changes in
hormonal areas, including no premenstrual symptoms and regular
cycles for the first time in thirty years! Our energy levels and overall
health have improved noticeably.*

Dicksey Higgins ~ Premenopause

*About three years ago I was experiencing all of the symptoms of
Premenopause: frequent headaches, irritability, sore breasts, bloating
and unbelievable "brain fog." I spent most afternoons napping. I did-
n't even care if I got up to make supper. I decided I needed some help,
but I wanted to avoid taking the standard estrogen replacements.*

*At this time a friend introduced me to the strategies for vibrant
health. After reading some information on the strategies I became excited to find out that they could help my body overcome the pain of*

*arthritis in my knees, shoulders, and hands. My joints hurt every time
I walked down stairs or on uneven ground.*

*In just a few days I noticed positive changes. For the first time in ten
years I felt an urge to take a walk! The worst of the PMS symptoms - -
the headaches, bloating and brain fog - - disappeared within a month.
No more naps, and I wake up each morning feeling refreshed.*

*Also, in four months I lost twenty-five pounds, and have kept them
off for nearly three years.*

*My entire family uses the strategies for vibrant health. We choose
preventative measures as opposed to disease management.*

Cameo Kempf ~ Depression, Candida Albicans (yeast problem)

*I believe my problems started to surface and snowball while I was in
college. My senior year 1994 is the time I can really point to when I
think about the beginning of not feeling 100 percent well. It wasn't
until 1996 that I hit absolute rock bottom and realized something was
wrong with me. I wanted to sleep all the time, I was nasty to people
when I was trying so hard to be nice, and I was very depressed. The
doctor I worked for prescribed pills and I got very ill. I knew deep
down he had to be wrong and began to look for a natural route.*

*My mom heard about strategies for health and the awesome testi-
monies of people we knew who had chronic fatigue and candida
problems. After four months before I began to notice signs of change,
my energy level started to rise and anxiety attacks were less intense. I
am even-tempered and can exercise without becoming totally exhausted,
and people began to notice my eyes looked clearer and more alert!
Overall, I am still healing but am being patient as my health and
well-being continue to improve.*

Lanette E. Passarelli ~ Epilepsy

*Thirty years ago, when I was eleven years old, I became a diabetic
and developed epilepsy. Over the years, along with insulin, I took
Dilentin and Phenobarbital to avoid having seizures. When I
was thirty they replaced the Dilentin and Phenobarbital with 600*

milligrams of Tegretol a day.

During my college years I had the hardest time with seizures, but later, as an adult, they became more sporadic. In 1982 an electroencephalogram (EEG) indicated I still had some neurological disorders. My doctor kept my medications the same.

In July 1997 a friend introduced me to the principles of vibrant health. In February 1999 I went to my neurologist for my annual check-up. (My last seizure was in 1994.) He suggested an EEG. Depending on what he found, I might be able to stop taking the Tegretol. To make a long story short, the EEG showed no signs of epilepsy and I was gradually weaned from the Tegretol. Within eighteen months I was free from any signs of epilepsy and two years later I am off Tegretol!

I never thought I would see the day when my body would heal itself. I know one day I'll be off insulin!

Diane Mueller ~ Multiple Sclerosis

I was diagnosed with multiple sclerosis in November 1997. I began taking 60 milligrams of Prednisone for double vision. I did not like taking Prednisone as it wiped out my immune system, and made me feel sick and grouchy. When I started to taper off the Prednisone I went to my primary care doctor who suggested I try the strategies for vibrant health. (At the time I had not done any research on Multiple Sclerosis. I was in complete denial.) After trying the strategies, I no longer take Prednisone and show no signs of Multiple Sclerosis. (After learning more about the disease, I realized I probably had Multiple Sclerosis for fifteen years before I was diagnosed.)

Also, for years I had suffered from severe premenstrual syndrome. After three months on the product, I no longer cry over nothing or act like the Wicked Witch of the West. Thanks to the strategies for health I can now say the nightmare is over.

Helen Swayne ~ Macular Degeneration

About three-and-a-half years ago I was diagnosed with macular degeneration. At the time I was told I would probably go blind. There was nothing that could be done. To read normal print I had to use a magnifying glass.

My good friend introduced me to the strategies for vibrant health. Her husband had experienced success for his macular degeneration. I tried the strategies in February 1999. Within six weeks I noticed I could read without using the magnifying glass. There has been no negative change in my eyesight. It feels good to see! I also notice that my general health is much better.

Marlene and Winston Statham ~Child with Neuroaxonal Dystropy

In 1987 at the age of fifteen, our daughter Darcie started to experience a lot of health problems. She had headaches, then numbness in her arms and legs, mood changes, difficulty talking, and falling down. By the time she was eighteen she had deteriorated so much she was in a wheel chair. Her muscles were so weak she could not even turn herself over in bed. Actually, the only part of her body she could move at her will was her eyes. She was diagnosed with neuroaxonal dystrophy, a rare degenerative disease.

In May 1997 we tried the strategies for health with Darcie. After only a month she was able to wipe her face with her hand. In October 1997 she was able to print a letter of the alphabet on a piece of paper. By the spring of 1998 Darcie had gained quite a bit of control of her right hand. She could print her name in one-inch high letters and she started painting crafts. Also, she could sit up straighter and did not need her head support.

By the fall of 1998, she could print sentences on a page, staying in the lines. And by the end of 1998 Darcie could feed herself a complete meal and choking was much less frequent.

In the spring of 1999 Darcie could clap her hands together! In May 1999 she had total control of her bladder and bowel function, which meant the end of diapers. In June 1999 she took six steps between parallel bars and could support her whole weight. She has physiotherapy daily, so her movement continues to increase. She drools much less, is able to move her tongue from side to side, and is able to make some sounds. Additionally, she can now concentrate enough to read lots of books. We believe the discovery of these strategies is a gift from God.

Cameron Clark ~ High Cholesterol/Depression

In October 1996 I was diagnosed with serious clinical depression and spent the next year and a half on anti-depressants. Finally I was able to get off the antidepressants. I was anxious to be rid of the adverse side effects. Then, I was diagnosed with extremely high cholesterol. I was told I'd have to be on a cholesterol-lowering drug for the rest of my life. (I was in my thirties).

By June 1998 I had three major health concerns: how to reduce my risk of getting multiple sclerosis (my dad was diagnosed with Multiple Sclerosis in 1995), how to keep off anti-depressants, and how to control my cholesterol without dangerous side effects.

A friend introduced me to the principles of vibrant health. I soon noticed some changes. I had more energy, fewer colds, and lost some weight. And I started waking up refreshed and ready to face each day.

Today I am not depressed and I don't need to take antidepressants. Multiple Sclerosis no longer frightens me, because I've seen the research on how the better health strategies prevent it by giving the immune system the tools it needs to work properly. And, my cholesterol is well within a safe range.

Andrew & Cynthia Finley ~ son with severe migraines

Our son, Joshua, had suffered with severe migraine headaches for close to eight years. He would have, on the average, five to eight of these intense headaches each month. He would miss many days at school and other activities that many children get to enjoy during childhood. We seemed to try everything, but nothing worked. We even went to the head pediatric neurologist at New York University Medical Center, and his only solution was to keep Joshua from eating certain foods or using toxic drugs with side affects.

In January 1997 we were introduced to the strategies for health by a friend. Joshua has been using them for two and a half years now and we're happy to say that he has not had one headache since the day he started using them.

Debbi Scott ~ Chronic Depression

I am forty years old and since the age of nineteen I have been hospitalized five times for chronic depression. I did not want to live. I hated life. Many times I tried to end my life. I tried to cover my mental pain with prescription or street drugs. I can remember being depressed since the age of five.

My depression caused many physical problems. I had medication for everything. I had ulcers, gall bladder trouble, irritable bowel syndrome, panic attacks and esophagitis. I had a hysterectomy when I was twenty-one. Needless to say, I felt like crap all the time!

Sometime in 1994 my cousin from Seattle told me she had something she wanted me to try. At first I was not interested - - but she called me every day for a week. I promised to try the strategies for health for at least a month. After about three weeks I noticed a change - - and I actually took myself off all my medications. I started feeling better. Sure, I might have a bad day once in awhile - - but for the most part all of the problems I listed are gone!

5

INVISIBLE ASSASSINS
(The Metal Dynamic)

Dangerous Toxins

Foreign Invasion

Drinking Poisons

Sweet Seduction

Sweet Deception

Toxic Waste Dumps In Your Mouth

What Can You Do?

Trains Avoid Rocks

Miracle Stories

Dangerous Toxins

The third strategy to vibrant health and longevity is represented by the Metal dynamic. Metal is toxic. It is a foreign substance to your body, whether it is in large pieces such as bullets or in invisible microscopic amounts.

This strategy is about three things: **awareness, avoidance** and **reduction** of all toxic and foreign substances, which includes heavy metals and chemicals from the environment, as well as chemicals in food and all chemically *altered* foods that are toxic to the body. These toxins are very serious "stress checks" against your health account.

In ancient times, poison was put in food only if someone hated someone and wanted that person dead. In our modern era, the motivation is different, but with the same results. Today the motivation is money, combined with an indifference or refusal to put safety and human life above profit.

Examples of this include additives, pesticides, preservatives, coloring agents, hydrogenated oil, refined sugar and artificial sweeteners, such as aspartame (also known as NutraSweet).

There are two basic types of toxins: domestic and foreign. Domestic toxins are natural and are produced in the body as part of the normal process of life, similar to how ashes are a natural waste product from the burning of wood. Ideally, these are either neutralized and broken down in the body or expelled through the organs of elimination, such as the lungs, skin, kidneys, liver and bowels. Our body was designed to handle these internally produced toxins fairly easily.

Foreign Invasion

However, the foreign toxins that are introduced from outside the body add a significant and unintended burden to these organs of elimination. Foreign toxins can *severely* interfere with the immune and endocrine (hormones) systems.

For the most part, these foreign toxins are either natural substances that have been so severely altered as to become toxic, or man-made synthetic chemicals. In either case, they enter our bodies through three sources: the air we breathe, the water we drink and the food we eat. Research shows that there are between 300 and 500 toxins in our tissues today that were never found in the tissues of anyone before 1940. In fact, even the air at the North Pole is polluted with dioxin, one of the worst air pollutants and cancer causing agents. You are breathing dioxin right now and hundreds of other chemicals that you cannot taste, see or smell.

You can run, but you can not hide! Even our homes are not safe! In fact, according to the <u>Scientific American Magazine</u>, the February issue of 1998, our homes are even more dangerous than the "fresh" air outside, because the concentration of *toxins in the home is 300-500 percent HIGHER than outdoors!* A large part of how this occurs is from "outgas" which is the leaking of toxic chemicals from carpeting, pressed wood, detergents, household cleaners, ink, adhesives, glues, paints, dry cleaned clothes and pesticides. Recently, NASA discovered that plants like English Ivy, philodendrons, chrysanthemums, and spider plants will absorb many contaminants. Also using an ozone and negative ion generator can help neutralize much of your indoor air pollutants.

And it can start early! Industrial chemicals and pesticides are even present in the amniotic fluid surrounding fetuses. In tests done on 53 pregnant women, researchers found that ONE-THIRD of their future offspring were being exposed in the womb to DDE—a by-product of the deadly pesticide DDT, which has been banned in the US since 1972. Industrial chemicals such as polychorinated biphenyls and the by-products of the pesticide lindane have also invaded the womb.

Is Your Child Being Poisoned?

Consumer's Union, publisher of <u>CONSUMER REPORTS</u> magazine announced in February of 1999 that many U.S. fruits and vegetables carry pesticide residues that exceed the limits that EPA considers safe for children. *"Using U.S. Department of Agriculture statistics based on 27,000 food samples from 1994 to 1997, the magazine looked at foods children are most likely to eat,"* the NEW YORK TIMES reported. *"Almost all the foods tested for pesticide residues were within legal limits, but were frequently well above the levels the Environmental Protection Agency says are safe for young children."* According to the Consumer's Union Report, even one serving of some fruits and vegetables can exceed safe daily limits for young children the TIMES reported.

"Methyl parathion accounts for most of the total toxicity on the foods that were analyzed, particularly peaches, frozen and canned green beans, pears and apples. Late last year [EPA] said that methyl parathion posed an 'unacceptable risk' but that it had not taken any action to ban it or reduce its use. Organophosphates [such as methyl parathion] are <u>neurological poisons</u> and work the same on humans as they do on insects," the NEW YORK TIMES said.

Immune System in Free Fall!

The increase of toxins in our environment and food is believed by many scientists and researchers to be the PRIMARY cause in the decline of our immune system function.

In fact, according to measurements done by various medical researchers over the years, our natural killer cells (the most active part of our immune system, and the first line of defense against bacteria, viruses or cancer), declined by an average of 1 percent a year between 1981 and 1991; but from 1991 to 1997, the average drop tripled to 3 percent a year! **This is a 29 percent drop in just sixteen years — and this decline appears to be accelerating!**

What can you do? The most important thing is to *commit right now* to do all you can, since your health and your life depend upon it. I suggest a three-fold strategy: awareness, avoidance, and reduction of the toxins already in your system.

What You Don't Know Can Hurt You!

First, before you can *avoid* toxins, you need to be *aware* of them.

Awareness is your first strategy. Start by investing the time to read the labels on everything you buy. If it contains any non-food substances or chemicals, DON'T put it in your body (if you care about your health)! If you don't know what something is on a label, the chances are that it is not good for you. Why pay money to poison yourself?

Just because the negative effect is not immediate does not mean it isn't damaging and robbing you of your health! And the negative effect can accumulate and not show up for years.

For example, do not use over-the-counter medicines casually, including remedies for allergies, colds, pain, heartburn and headaches. Remember, what percentage of drugs are toxic? That's right—100 percent. Save them, and antibiotics, for a major crisis, not for minor things. In fact, aspirin according to one medical researcher, causes bleeding in the stomach 100 percent of the time.

Drugs on Tap!

Furthermore, you are getting too many drugs *already* on a daily basis if you drink tap water! Because 90 percent of drugs are excreted by the body through the urine, and most water is recycled, they end up in the tap water. This alarming discovery was first made in Germany in 1998. *When American tap water was checked, the concentration of antibiotics was a 1000 percent higher than in the Germany water!*

Plus, over half of the antibiotics produced in the U.S. are fed to cattle and poultry which is then eaten by us. No wonder antibiotics are less and less effective when they are really needed. In the mean time, getting them in our food and water adds more stress to your internal organs and systems!

Toxic Oil in your Favorite Foods!

One common substance that many people *assume* (out of ignorance) is okay is partially hydrogenated oil, which is a form of "trans oil." This dangerous stuff is in numerous processed foods, including and especially margarine. According to Dr. Sheldon Deal, it takes the body 55 days to get rid of the hydrogenated oil from just ONE potato chip.

Don't you think your body has better ways to expend its energy? If you knew the whole truth, you would avoid margarine and any other foods with partially hydrogenated oil just like you would avoid a food with axle grease mixed in — regardless of how good it may look or taste. Partially hydrogenated oil is a MAJOR "stress check" you don't want to be writing against your health account.

DRINKING POISON

Would you volunteer to drink something with poison if you were offered enough money? What if it was diluted enough that the effect was delayed for years? Wouldn't the only reason you'd do such a thing is if you lacked the knowledge?

Two important poisons (and toxins) to avoid are chlorine and fluoride. Some very convincing research indicates that chlorine may be a primary cause of the buildup of cholesterol in arteries. Chlorine irritates and damages the arterial linings, which the body then patches up with cholesterol. It has been linked to both heart disease and cancer.

During World War I, guess what was used to kill hundreds of thousands of people? Clorine gas, which is a deadly poison! For this reason, the people in Western Europe are pretty sensitive about chlorine. So ozone and ultraviolet light is used instead of chlorine in water.

According to Dr. Joseph Price, M.D.,

"Chlorine is the greatest crippler and killer of modern times; it is an insidious poison…we thought we were preventing epidemics of one disease, but we were creating another."

Use purified or better yet, *revitalized* water—your body and life deserves it! (See the Appendix for information on revitalized water).

SWEET SEDUCTION

Not all toxins are synthetic chemicals. Food that start off as good and natural can be so severely *altered* as to become toxic, yet have the appearance of being good, much like the deceptive "gift" of the Trojan horse of ancient history.

The most destructive "Trojan horse" of modern times is white sugar. *Having been stripped of all nutritive value, refined white sugar is a virtual anti-nutrient or nutritional "black hole" that robs your body of existing nutrients just to handle the sugar it gets.* It is your most dangerous enemy, having so thoroughly infiltrated both our food supply and our culture.

Can something that tastes so good be so bad? In medical literature, over 60 ailments, including heart disease, cancer and diabetes have been linked to the use of sugar.

White sugar is extremely seductive. It seduces us through the pleasure we get from our taste buds. Three thousand years ago, King Solomon described a similar kind of seduction in his graphic narrative of a naïve young man being seduced by a prostitute:

"Soon she has him eating out of her hand, bewitched by her honeyed speech. Before you know it, he's trotting behind her, like a calf led to the butcher shop, like a stag lured into ambush and then shot with an arrow; like a bird flying into a net not knowing that its flying life is over.

"So friends, listen to me, take these words seriously. Don't fool around with a woman like that; don't even stroll through her neighborhood. Countless victims come under her spell; she's the death of many a poor man. She runs a halfway house to hell, fits you out with a shroud and a coffin." Proverbs 7 (The Message version).

Everyone's Doing it

In every culture studied, the pattern has been that degenerative diseases, such as "the 95 percent," have risen as the use of sugar has increased. According to Dr. Cleave, it takes about 20 years after the introduction of sugar and white flour for a culture to go from virtually no disease to having the degenerative diseases so common in the Western world.

Two hundred years ago, sugar consumption was less than 20 pounds per year per person. It more than tripled by 1900. Now it's up to 152 pounds of sugar each year for the average American! Dr. Frederick Banting, who won the Nobel Prize for his insulin-extraction method, found that the number of diabetes cases in the United States increased proportionately with the per-capita consumption of sugar.

White flour and other high glycemic index foods (to be explained in Chapter Seven) can be just as bad as white sugar, because they are quickly broken down into sugar. Not only does this stress your immune system, but to add insult to injury, half of any refined carbohydrate can be converted to fat, which certainly doesn't make you look good!

Sugar in any form, including refined carbohydrates (white flour based food such as bread and pasta) and especially in soda pop, can be a major "stress check" against your health account. Even too much natural sugar in the form of a large glass of fruit juice or a lot of fruit at one sitting (especially high glycemic fruit like raisins and ripe bananas), can stress your pancreas and reduce the ability of your white blood cells to kill germs up to five hours after consumption.

<u>SWEET DECEPTION</u>

In a commendable but misguided effort to escape the dangers of sugar, people have flocked to artificial sweeteners, thinking they can "have their cake and eat it, too." However, you can't fool mother nature nor your body. Research now indicates that artificial sweeteners are even *more* harmful than the altered sweeteners (sugar).

The truth about aspartame's toxicity is far different than what the NutraSweet Company would have you believe. In February of 1994, the U.S. Department of Health and Human Services released a list of adverse reactions reported to the FDA (DHHS 1994). **Aspartame accounted for more than 75 percent of all adverse reactions reported to the FDA's Adverse Reaction Monitoring System (ARMS).**

Here are just some of the reactions by humans to aspartame: abdominal pain, anxiety attacks, arthritis, asthma, atrophied testes, edema (fluid retention), blood sugar control problems, brain cancer (pre-approval studies in animals), breathing difficulties, can't think straight, chest pains, chronic fatigue, death, depression, headaches and migraines, dizziness, heart palpitations, hypertension (high blood pressure), impotency and sexual problems, inability to concentrate, insomnia, irritability, joint pains, "marked personality changes," memory loss, menstrual problems, migraines and severe headaches, panic attacks, phobias, rashes, seizures and convulsions, slurring of speech, tachycardia, tremors, vision loss, and weight gain. In 1995 the FDA admitted to 10,000 complaints.

Have you ever had any of these symptoms? One neurologist stated: *"If we had had the facts on what aspartame causes there would be a lot of patients alive today."* And world famous toxicologist, Dr. George Schwartz, has already written a research paper on aspartame escalating breast and prostate cancer

---

Soda pop may taste good, but the artificial chemicals in soda are like beating your liver with a chemical baseball bat. And for that you pay a heavy price.

Over time, artificial sweeteners are a very serious "stress check" against your health account and will lower your balance considerably.

For a wealth of valuable references on aspartame, visit www.dorway.com, www.presidiotex.com/aspartame/ and http://web2.airmail.net/marystod.

TOXIC WASTE DUMPS IN YOUR MOUTH

Would you feel comfortable living close to a toxic waste dump? How about having it in your house? *What if it were in your mouth?* That's exactly what has happened to millions of Americans. The so-called safe fillings called amalgam (known as "silver" fillings) contain a very toxic heavy metal called mercury. Every time you chew, mercury vapors are released that are devastating to your immune system and other tissues, especially your brain. Many serious conditions have been linked to mercury in the mouth. I have chosen to have all mine removed, and you may want to do the same.

For more information, read "It's All In Your Head—The Link Between Mercury Amalgams and Illness" by Dr. Hal Huggins, or go to www.Hugnet.com or do a search on "amalgam" on the internet.

WHAT CAN YOU DO?

The third strategy in dealing with toxins (after awareness and avoidance) is to *reduce and get rid of toxins you've been storing in your tissues.* An essential part of this third strategy is drinking one quart of uncontaminated (purified) water every day for every 50 pounds of weight. Think about it—how clean would your clothes get if you tried to wash them with only a couple cups of water? Each glass of water is a nice deposit into your health account. Additional strategies for moving out toxins will be disclosed in the next chapter.

Regeneration Time

Another essential thing is to make sure you get enough "regeneration" time on a regular basis. "Regeneration" time is sleep.

The American Cancer Society did a massive six year study on a million Americans. The researchers found that those who slept less than seven hours a night were more likely to be dead in six years, and the same was true for those who slept more than ten hours a night. According to William Dement, M.D., who founded the world's first known sleep disorder at Stanford University, years of research indicate that people need to sleep one hour for every two hours they are awake, and that those who sleep about eight hours a day tend to live longer. Research seems to support that if you accumulate a sleep debt (averaging less than this), you are probably doing damage to your health and reducing your longevity. Plus, much of the detoxification occurs while you sleep, if you get enough! For more information on how to assess your sleep debt, go to www.sleepnet.com.

A "Phyto" a Day Keeps the Cancer Away

According to the American Institute of Cancer Research, "...*a wide variety of phytochemicals, protective substances found in vegetables and fruit, interact in the body to decrease risk of cancer and other illnesses such as diabetes and heart disease.*"

The National Cancer Institute recommends that we eat *five to seven* servings a day of fruits and vegetables (preferably vine ripened). They are a powerful source of anti-cancer and immune supporting phytochemicals (plant nutrients), which are wonderful deposits to make into your health account every day.

For valuable **FREE** information from the American Institute for Cancer Research, call (800) 843-8114 and request, "Taking a Closer Look at Phytochemicals—New Cancer Research" or visit their excellent web site at www.aicr.org.

If you are not eating five to seven servings a day of fruit and vegetables as recommended by the National Cancer Institute, I strongly recommend that you do what I did: find a phytochemical supplement to make up the difference. Besides the antioxidant benefits, this can also support your liver's detoxification. This can be an extremely important deposit into your health account.

Be sure to use a formula that has been proven scientifically to raise glutothione levels, which is the most powerful and important antioxidant. This is especially important to take if you eat fish, which, though a good food, tend to contain very high amounts of dangerous chemical pollutants. Shell and bottom feeding fish are the worst.

Detoxification with Acupressure

There is an indicator reflex point you can check yourself that may show a level of toxicity in your body. It is the fourth Acupuncture point on the Large Intestine Acupuncture Meridian. It is on your hands, located inside the junction (a "V" shape) formed by the bones from your thumb and index finger. Test for tenderness by massaging as hard as you can with your thumb and index finger (from the other hand, or have someone else do it).

Place your thumb on the top part of the hand in that wedge (about one inch from the third joint on the index finger and one inch from the second thumb joint). Place your index finger on the palm side, and squeeze that index finger and thumb together in a vigorous massaging motion.

The more tender that spot is, the more toxicity overload your body is dealing with. It should have zero pain at even the highest pressure. If it is tender, you can help your body reduce toxicity by massaging that point throughout the day for several days until the pain is gone. Doing this also stimulates your immune system according to Dr. Sheldon Deal. Doing this can be another important deposit into your health account.

You can also use this point to reduce or eliminate pain, including headaches and backaches, usually within twenty to thirty seconds.

For a wealth of additional invaluable information on how to identify and remove toxins, read <u>How To Stay Young and Healthy In A Toxic World</u>, by Ann Louise Gittleman.

You can also visit <u>www.scorecard.org</u> to discover what level of environmental toxins are in your area by zip code.

TRAINS AVOID ROCKS

This third strategy, based on the Metal dynamic, has to do with toxins that interfere with normal body functions and thus your health. Let's build a little further on the train analogy to give you some further insight into how the Metal dynamic applies to your health.

For your train to have a successful trip, you also must be careful to avoid any rocks and boulders that may fall on the tracks. Especially watch out for rock slides! And even the accumulative effect of a lot of small rocks, like pebbles and sand, will interfere with your journey. Ancient wisdom tells us to *"cleanse ourselves from every defilement (toxin) of flesh and spirit...."* (II Cor. 7:1b) and *"lay aside every encumbrance (heavy weights)...and run with endurance the race set before us."* (Hebrews 12:1b).

So just being on the right track (purpose—Fire dynamic), and being well-connected (Earth dynamic) to the tracks, other cars and your crew are not enough. You've got to keep your guard up for the dangers in the Metal dynamic.

Miracle Stories

Sharon Graham ~ Chemically Poisoned

I was chemically poisoned in 1985 by new building materials. My immune system was severely damaged, and nearly destroyed. I literally became allergic to everything. I could no longer go anywhere, and no one could visit me. When my husband would come home from work, he would have to undress in the garage, go to the basement and take a shower and change his clothing before he could come into the house where I was. I could no longer use anything plastic. Food had to be stored in glass and cellophane. Gone, of course, were all household cleaners, detergents, shampoos, hair conditioner, hair spray, nail polish, and makeup. I could no longer wear any clothing made with synthetic fibers. Most of my clothes had to be given away. The only lifeline I had was the telephone, and I quickly became allergic to the plastic on that. My husband bought a speakerphone (long before they were popu-

lar) which became my only connection to the outside world. I couldn't even walk down the street because the clothes-dryer vents were often spewing out detergent and fabric softener fumes.

My body was overloaded with toxins. I quickly became allergic to almost all foods. I was extremely ill, and we had very little hope for a number of years. My initial symptoms were almost continual headaches, which became increasingly more and more severe. Memory loss, inability to organize my thoughts, and irritability accompanied the headaches. I developed severe joint pain, which eventually was diagnosed as arthritis. Muscle aches, weakness, fatigue, low-grade fever, and constant flu-like symptoms were also present. Digestive problems developed from the leaky-gut syndrome. Due to my nursing background, I thought I had either multiple sclerosis or lupus. I also knew that my symptoms were so bizarre that a physician would only say, "It's all in your head." My body was on a rapid, downhill spiral.

I've spent the last twelve years fighting to regain my health. I've tried many, many products. I've gone to many different types of health-care practitioners, and I've tried numerous dietary regimes. I had regained about 50 percent to 60 percent of my health a few years ago as a result of having undertaken a serious detoxification process which included large quantities of high quality dietary supplementation along with fresh vegetable juices, consistent exercise, and eating almost all organically grown food. Finally, at least I didn't feel sick all of the time. And I was gradually able to be out and about more. A few years ago, the addition of some "green superfood" also increased my sense of well being, but my immune system still had a long way to go.

Truthfully, I had heard about one of these strategies for health in 1996, but I also heard doctors and scientists developed it. I know that may be a drawing card for many, but to me it was a very big turn-off. After all, what did they know? They had contributed toward my ill-health years ago. Therefore, I never gave the strategies a second look until a year and a half later when our friend and neighbor was helped tremendously with ulcerative colitis after trying them.

I slowly and very skeptically began trying them, and soon began experiencing a healing crisis. My body continues to go through some tremendous and exciting changes, all for the better. My improvements are profound and incredible. I now look healthy and vibrant! I am able to do many things that most people take for granted. Things like going shopping at the local mall or meeting a friend for lunch at a restaurant. I can now run errands for my husband, go to the post office to mail a package, visit a neighbor in her home, and attend church without being ill for days afterwards. Recently, I was even able to fly to Colorado Springs with my husband when he had to travel there to attend a class. These strategies have truly changed my life.

Eugene Fox ~ Chronic Bowel Disease/Arthritis

I was sixty-three and my wife was fifty-one when we were first intro-duced to the principles of vibrant health and longevity. Generally we enjoyed good health, except I had chronic bowel disease and my wife had arthritis in her hands, which was threatening to stop her from working as a healthcare aide.

We started the principles because we were convinced they would be good for our health - - but we did not anticipate any great changes. Well, in three weeks my bowel disease cleared up and has not returned. In four months the arthritis in my wife's hands was 95 percent gone. We have enjoyed other benefits since then - - with more to come, no doubt!

Chuck Deetjen ~ Benign Prostate Hyperplasia

For the past four or five years I have been faced with waking up three, four, and five times a night to go to the bathroom. This is not terribly uncommon in older men who suffer from an enlarged prostate gland. The disease is known as benign prostate hyperplasia. It results in a restricted flow and retention of urine in the bladder. It is uncomfort-able and I felt tired due to the sleep interruption.

For the last two years I have been on a drug called Flomax which helps some. In January of 1999 my urologist suggested I have laser surgery to give me relief. I asked on the Internet if anyone had such surgery and was told "DON'T HAVE SURGERY".

I started using the strategies for vibrant health that I learned about from a friend. After about three months I started sleeping five or six hours a night. What a blessing!

Chris Lecce ~ Child with ADD/ADHD

Our son Dustin was diagnosed with ADHD (Attention Deficit Hyperactivity Disorder) in 1992. He had been on a full range of drugs that are easily administered for ADHD. Currently he was on Dexedrine. Of course, he suffered from numerous side effects: loss of appetite, restless sleep, fatigue, rapid weight loss, etc. We were tired of these medications and the varying dosages his doctors prescribed.

So we took Dustin off the Dexedrine and tried the strategies for vibrant health. What a difference! His appetite returned, he tuned into his family, and his energy level balanced out. Also, his school grades improved. Instead of earning C's, D's and F's, he earns A's, B's, and C's. We are truly thankful for these strategies.

Ettor J. Strada ~ Gulf War Syndrome

I am a Gulf War veteran and I have had many of the symptoms of Gulf War syndrome. Some of those ailments include: headaches, severe fatigue, aching joints, sore muscles, memory loss, abdominal pain, huge bleeding boils, severe nausea, and severe mood swings.

Before I started the strategies to health I was not very happy with life. I was not suicidal, but I was not much fun to be around. I did not feel like doing anything. After I started the strategies a friend shared with me, I started feeling like a normal person again. I started having more fun with my family and actually wanted to go out and do things. I do not require as much sleep and always feel the drive and energy to do whatever I want to do.

Sue Whisenant ~ Sports Injury

Two years ago I turned my ankle while out walking and fell and broke my shoulder in two places. The doctor said I might need to have surgery to repair it. I was naturally filled with anxiety, and didn't want any surgery.

My arm was put in a sling and I was sent home with Demerol for the pain. I really didn't want to take the Demerol, but the pain was intense. It relieved the pain for a few hours, but made me sick.

*A friend shared the strategies for health with me and I decided to
try them.*

*In three weeks when I returned to the doctor to see if I needed
surgery, the x-rays showed the bones were healed and I was able to
raise my arm above my head. The doctor couldn't believe what he
was seeing. This resulted in my giving a seminar to his clinic staff
about the use of the strategies.*

Diane Davis ~ Pulmonary Hypertension

*Seven years ago I was diagnosed with a rare condition called
pulmonary hypertension. I got the condition because my chemistry
changed after a simple hernia surgery. I began throwing blood clots
to my lungs.*

*It went untreated for two years. My symptoms were shortness of
breath and lack of energy. I finally got sick enough to find a pulmonary doctor. After some testing I was told I needed an open-lung
biopsy to make sure I did indeed have this condition. They removed my
lower left lobe because it was so full of blood clots. The surgery was
very painful and I had to be in the intensive-care unit for three days.*

*Then depression set in and I was getting worse. The doctor's only
solution was to give me an antidepressant, which gave no relief. My
activities were restricted because of the oxygen tank I carried under my
clothes, and my grandbabies were scared of me because of the canula
on my face.*

*I had severe setbacks with the blood clots and the side effects of
the blood thinner. With this lung condition comes many medical
problems, not just blood clots but upper respiratory infections and
stomach problems.*

*The answer came in the form of my soon to be son-in-law. He heard
of these strategies for health and longevity and wanted me to try them.
Since then two years have passed and I have become a walking miracle. The oxygen use is only at night and I am off all medications except
my blood thinner. I don't have stomach problems, upper respiratory
infections, or depression and I feel wonderful.*

*My last checkup was last week. I had a breathing test and it was the
best ever. The doctor just smiled and said, "You are truly blessed." I*

know I am, but without the help of God and the information my son-in-law gave me I don't think I would be here today.

Angie Nanos ~ Severe Muscle Spasms

I had spent several months in tears. I was unable to sit for more than a few minutes at a time, and I was uncomfortable standing. I couldn't lie down without crying because of severe muscle spasms. I had become 75 to 85 percent bedridden.

I found out that I had two slipped discs in my neck and a degenerating spine with several destroyed discs in my lower back. My symptoms were constant pain in my legs, arms, and neck. I had almost constant muscle spasms, and suffered numbness in my legs, feet, arms, and hands. With this, I suffered severe burning in my hands, feet, and ears. I had extreme fatigue and weakness.

The doctors told me that I should put off surgery for as long as possible because I already had one fusion in my neck and I would require surgeries throughout my lifetime. I found myself very discouraged, lonely, and depressed.

I am a single mother with two teenage daughters, who became very angry because I was not available for their needs. One night I was on the Internet and I received a message from a woman. We struck up a conversation, which lead us into talking for several days. My life hasn't been the same since.

I tried the strategies to vibrant health and longevity and after two weeks I realized how much better I was feeling. By the third week I was no longer taking pain medication or muscle relaxants. I was out of bed and felt as though I had been set free.

I no longer feel desperate to find someone to care for my children, I do that myself. I have gone from pain and suffering, discouragement and desperation, to health, strength, and fullness of life.

Treva House ~ Migraine Headaches and Ulcers

Migraine headaches and acid stomach problems (ulcers) were very common in my dad's family. I remember it was such a sad day, when at age eleven, I had my first migraine. It was sad for the entire family because the younger a person is with their first migraine, the more severe it often is.

For more than forty years I suffered with CONSTANT headaches - ranging from mild to very severe. Five or six times a year my head would hurt so bad and so long that it would still be sore once I got some relief. Because it was well known in my family that going to the doctor for pain medications for migraines led to worsening of our stomach problems, and didn't help much with the headaches, I refused medical diagnosis or treatment.

In 1995 I tried the strategies for vibrant health because a friend told me about them. Because of the improvement my husband and I saw within a few weeks, the strategies soon were routine.

I continued to see improvements with my headaches and stomach problems. Soon I noticed significant improvements in my knee and muscle aches, severe chronic sinus condition, and general fatigue. Even after several months, I wake up hardly able to comprehend that I am still pain free. The best part is I am also healthier than I have ever been.

Jacqueline Copeland ~ Nerve Repair
Our story is just beginning. Our youngest daughter was born November 12, 1997 just after her twin brother. She was exposed to a virus before she was born called CMV, which damaged the nerves in her ears. She was profoundly deaf and scheduled to receive a cochlear implant...that is until a friend shared one of the strategies for better health.

After four months of these health principles, we have started to see improvement in her hearing. In fact, she has regained a quarter of her hearing in just four and a half months. All the doctors have told us that nerves that are damaged just cannot heal, but we know differently. Given the right strategy our bodies can heal themselves. Now at twenty months she is able to hear sounds and is beginning to say her first words. The therapists that work with her every week are stunned.

Darsie Strome ~ Clinical Depression
I suffered from clinical depression for years. I felt depressed, anxious,

and fatigued, even when I was taking antidepressants. I have been on at least five different medications.

A friend shared the strategies for vibrant health with me. Within a month I wasn't fatigued, something that had plagued me since childhood. Due to severe side effects, it took me three months to wean myself off of the antidepressant Efexor. I am completely off the antidepressant - - and I feel great!

Evelyn Daugherty ~ daughter with uncontrollable seizures (Sturge Weber Syndrome)

My daughter, Mary Daugherty, who is now in her forties, was diagnosed at five weeks of age with Sturge Weber syndrome, a rare disease that affected the left side of her head, from the center of the face to the center of the back of her head. There was a massive, vascular, intercranial tumor that involved the nervous system. At that time it was treated with massive doses of radiation, the only known treatment.

The disease is progressive; it accelerates the aging process and slowly destroys the brain cells. In late 1996, she was diagnosed with uncontrollable seizures, which is a normal part of the disease.

I started using the health strategies in February 1997 after a friend shared them with me. After remarkable improvement in my health, we decided to try them with Mary. The change was significant. She had fewer seizures and since November 1997 to present, she has been seizure-free!

This is not all. She's grown hair back where she lost it because of the radiation treatments. She's reading again and walking with her dad at the mall.

Lisa Seatter ~ Endometriosis and Grave's disease

When I was seventeen I was at a time in my life when I should not have had to worry about my health, or so I thought.

Then one night I woke in the middle of the night to excruciating pain in my lower abdomen. It was so painful that I thought someone was stabbing me in the stomach. I was rushed to the hospital and was kept overnight thinking it was my appendix. After laparoscopic surgery I was diagnosed with endometriosis.

I was to go in for some exploratory knee surgery a few months later. I happened to go to a chiropractor just before my physical and he mentioned I should get my thyroid checked out. When I was having my pre-operation physical I mentioned it to my doctor. I was immediately sent for testing, and a week later I was diagnosed with Grave's disease and put on thyroid medication.

After months of getting bad colds and other related illnesses, and a car accident where I suffered whiplash, my parents began to encourage me to try the strategies for vibrant health. When you are in a health crisis you have to try something. This included eating healthier foods and taking things out of my life such as pop and junk food. Within two months I was off ALL of my medications, including Ibuprofen, which I had been eating like candy. I was bored and looking for work again. It felt good to feel good. It had been a LONG time. Everything was back to normal. I am now twenty-three and life couldn't be better. I will not stop using the strategies.

Kim & Deidre Triffitt ~ Lennox Gasteau Syndrome & Autism

What do you do when a specialist tells you your eighteen month old son will never amount to anything physically or mentally, not to waste your time, energy, or money trying to help him as his health will get progressively worse and he will basically be a vegetable?

Of course we were devastated to hear that our son had Lennox Gasteau syndrome and autism. Our beautiful son Corom went from a happy, healthy, contented baby to a baby who cried continually and had seizures all day and night. He was only able to sleep one half hour at a time, as once he would get off to sleep he would be woken by yet another seizure.

Our life was turned upside down. At this stage we had two older sons, Levi & Jarom, and I was pregnant with our fourth child, Emily. We went on a frantic medical search to help our son. For six years we went to numerous doctors, specialists, therapists. We did our homework, spent thousands of dollars, made numerous trips overseas. We felt so helpless. Watching our son deteriorate day by day was the most painful experience we have ever had. Corom lost all his skills; he was like a stroke patient that had to be taught everything again.

At eight years old we started Corom on the strategies for vibrant health and longevity that a friend told us about. That week was the first time he took himself to the toilet. He had been toilet timed, but not toilet trained. His language and comprehension improved. He now sleeps eight to ten hours a night.

Previously he was continually getting colds, the flu, and infections. The only thing that helped relieve the symptoms was antibiotic injections, which we hated giving him. Now after four years of using the strategies, Corom has only had three minor colds, and health wise he is great.

6

MOVING FOR LIFE
(The Water Dynamic)

Movement

Water for Healing

Moving Toxins Out

Sweating It Out

Moving Your Whole Body

Bounce Your Way to Health

Little Wheelchairs

Moving Stuck Energy

Moving Toward Your Future

Trains Move Fast!

Miracle Stories

MOVEMENT

The fourth strategy to vibrant health and longevity is represented by the Water dynamic, which represents movement. Movement also supports your immune system's function. Movement is characteristic of fresh water, whereas motionless water is stagnant and becomes a source of trouble. In fact, when something stops moving, we conclude that it is dead, since movement is a basic sign of life. When your heart stops moving (beating), which means blood is not moving and delivering essential oxygen and nutrients to the cells, the "game is over." How can you insure adequate movement to maintain and enhance your life and health?

WATER FOR HEALING

Water is the most essential component for internal movement and chemical processes, including the daily cleansing processes through the kidneys, bowels and skin. According to F. Batmanghelidj, M.D., long-term insufficiency of water (chronic dehydration) is the root cause of most major degenerative diseases in our country.

Dr. Batmanghelidj wrote a shocking milestone book, _Your Body's Many Cries for Water—You are not Sick, You are Thirsty,_ which is based on astounding original research and supported by hundreds of medical articles. In this incredible book, he presents a very convincing and scientifically based case that chronic dehydration is the primary causative factor in asthma, allergies, depression, diabetes, rheumatoid arthritis, high blood pressure, high cholesterol, anginal pain, cancer, ulcers, colitis, headaches and backaches!

As outrageous as this initially sounds, his research and conclusions are being supported by other doctors, such as Barry Kendler, Ph.D., Adjunct Faculty member of the Graduate Nutrition Program at the New York Medical College, who wrote,

"I had the opportunity of reading some of your publications concerning the significance of adequate hydration and the role of chronic dehydration in the etiology [cause] of disease. I carefully examined many of the references that you cited, especially those in your paper published in Anticancer Research (1987:7:971). Every reference I checked was properly used to support your hypothesis....I conclude, based upon study of your revolutionary concept, that its implementation by health care professionals and by the general public, is certain to have an enormous positive impact both on well being and on health care economics. Accordingly, I will do all that I can to publicize the importance of your findings."

For example, Dr. Batmanghelidj has personally treated over 3,000 patients with dyspeptic pain, with water only. In 100 percent of them, their clinical problems associated with the pain disappeared by just drinking enough water. This was reported in the Journal of Clinical Gastroenterology in June 1983.

Flush Those Cancer Cells Down the Toilet!

A recent study in the New England Journal of Medicine is the first to demonstrate a clear link between increased liquid intake and decreased bladder cancer of the two types most commonly found in developed countries: papillary and flat transitional cell carcinomas.

The study looked at the eating, drinking, exercise and smoking habits of 47,909 American men from 1986 to early 1996.

Men who drank at least six glasses of water a day cut their risk of bladder cancer in half compared with men who had less than one glass, regardless of how much they drank in total liquids.

Besides water, no other beverage had an independent beneficial effect.

And because smoking greatly increases the quantity of carcinogens in urine, this study, like previous research, found that the risk of *bladder cancer was nearly four times higher among heavy smokers than it was among non-smokers.*

"The quality of what you drink may ... be as important as how much (or little) you imbibe," according to one researcher who evaluated this study. Because of the hundreds of toxic chemicals in water, it is imperative to drink only purified or better yet, revitalized water. For more information on revitalized or energized water as distinct from just "purified" water, read the section on revitalized water in the appendix.

Practical Tips for Drinking

Here are some practical tips you can use immediately to improve your health based on Dr. Batmanghelidj's research.

Do not *assume* that thirst is a reliable indicator of your need for water. It is NOT! The *absolute minimum* you need is six to eight 8-ounce glasses of water a day.

But don't settle for just the minimum any more than you would settle for minimum wage! Ideally, you need one quart per 50 pounds of weight.

Do not *assume* that other beverages, such as coffee, tea, juices, alcohol and soft drinks count as water, even though they are 99 percent water. The body processes these as food. In fact, soft drinks and caffeine-containing beverages have a *dehydrating* effect, and are "stress checks" against your health account. As a result, to counteract for this dehydrating effect, two glasses of water must be consumed for every bottle or can of soft drink or cup of coffee consumed to offset this dehydrating effect.

The best *time* to drink water is as follows: one or two glasses of water immediately upon rising in the morning; a glass one half hour *before* eating a meal, and a glass of water two and a half hours after each meal; and one or two glasses of water just before retiring. Keep drinking throughout the day, whether you are thirsty or not. Remember, every glass of water is a good deposit into your health account.

When you are under stress, you need more water. If you forget to drink your water a half hour before your meal, it's better to drink it anyway, even if it's right before you eat, rather than with your food.

Also, research is further indicating that *sipping* water gives your body much better usage of water than gulping. You will not get the full value of water if you gulp a lot of water at once. Sipping it throughout the day is much better.

MOVING TOXINS OUT

Another very important type of movement is your bowels. If your bowels are not moving easily two or three times a day (once per meal), you may be constipated, and reabsorbing toxins back into your bloodstream. You don't want to be literally "full of it!" A common expression among health practitioners is "death begins in the colon."

According to a study published in Epidemilogy by Emily White, Ph.D., professor of Epidemilogy at Washington University in Seattle, the chance of developing cancer of the colon is 400 percent more in those people who feel constipated at least once a week, than those who rarely or never experience constipation. Also, the people who use commercial laxatives were also at high risk.

Although constipation can have many causes, the most common is too little fiber and insufficient water. Make sure you eat seven servings a day of vegetables and fruit and drink at least eight glasses of water. I take extra fiber with my two glasses of water every morning, and just prior to going to bed. Consider using either psyllium seed husks or a more advanced fiber formula. You may want to have a colonic done twice a year as well.

SWEATING IT OUT

Another very important way your body was designed to move toxins out is through the largest organ of your body, your skin. As you perspire, toxins are carried out of your system. This is why hot baths and saunas can be so valuable to your health. Many people, influenced by advertising, are making the serious mistake of *blocking* this important outflow of toxins by using an antiperspirant, which is a serious "stress check." What would happen to your car if you stuck a banana in the tail pipe to block the exhaust?

Antiperspirant, as the name clearly indicates, prevents you from perspiring, thereby inhibiting the body from purging toxins from below the armpits. As a result, the toxins tend to accumulate in lymph nodes below the arms. This high concentration of toxins can lead to cell mutations, which can lead to CANCER. Nearly all breast cancer tumors occur in the upper outside quadrant of the breast area. This is precisely where the lymph nodes are located.

Men are less likely (but not completely exempt) to develop breast cancer prompted by antiperspirant usage because most of the antiperspirant product is caught in their hair and is not directly applied to the skin. Women who apply antiperspirant right after shaving increase the risk further because shaving causes almost imperceptible nicks in the skin which give the chemicals entrance into the body from the armpit area.

Regular deodorants are very suspect as well. Just look at all the chemicals in them — do you really want these in your body? Your body is less able to defend itself from chemicals that enter through the skin than if they had gone through the stomach and been handled by the liver.

Sweat is actually odorless. It's the bacteria growing in the sweat that causes the odor. If you wash, you don't need deodorants. I have not used them for 25 years and know many others who feel the same way.

MOVING YOUR WHOLE BODY

Unfortunately, most people don't really believe that physical activity is that important, or else they would do more of it. This is evident based on the fact that the average American adult spends 28 hours a week motionless in front of the TV (also known as the E.I.R.—Electronic Income Reducer!). Just as movement is a sign of life, a lack of movement is a sign that there is less life. When we refer to someone as "full of life," we are not thinking of someone who sits around or does not move much. A person who has vibrant health has a high physical activity level.

What is the price you pay for incorporating more physical activity in your life? The short-term *perceived* cost is that you will have less time to do other things.

But the experience of many people invalidates that misperception, because when you have adequate physical activity, you have more energy and are able to get more done more efficiently. Furthermore, you will actually end up having *more* time in the long run, since you are likely to live years or decades longer!

The real price that you should pay close attention to is what it will cost you to *not* invest some regular time into physical movement: death and disease. This is when the accumulation of "stress checks," of which lack of movement is one, puts you into permanent "health bankruptcy."

Move or Die!

As many as 12 percent of all deaths—250,000 per year (that's 685 deaths a day; one every two minutes)—in the U.S. may be attributed indirectly to a lack of regular physical activity according to the <u>Wellness Letter</u> published in association with the School of Public Health, University of California, Berkeley.

A Yale University study of more than 9,000 white male veterans, aged 50 to 60, showed that those who reported inactive lifestyles were nearly *seven times more likely to suffer a stroke* than men who were moderately or very active. A daily walk of only one mile was found to be the minimum activity for reducing stroke risk.

Regular physical movement is not just a good idea to keep in shape—it is *essential* to having vibrant health and longevity. If you knew that every hour of time you "saved" now, by not exercising, would cost you a day or week of your life later on, would you do anything differently?

In the February 1999 issue of <u>Harvard Heart</u>, the editors point out that *"...studies have shown that regular moderate exercise, such as brisk walking, is associated with a reduced risk for death from heart disease by one-third or more."*

Make Life a Moving Experience

How can you incorporate more physical movement into your life? First of all, decide that you will move more. Get a "clicker" that monitors how many steps you take each day. Get a cordless phone and walk as you talk—that's what I do. Walk up and down stairs whenever you have an opportunity. Living in a house without stairs seems to me to be a real disadvantage. Deliberately park your car farther away so you get to walk more. For an extra bonus, walk in the sunlight whenever possible because sunlight, as a health deposit, helps detoxify your body as well as create Vitamin D. It only takes about three to four minutes of sunlight for your body to make enough Vitamin D. Of course, too much sun is damaging and is a "stress check."

BOUNCE YOUR WAY TO HEALTH

In addition to walking, I do three other activities that I strongly recommend to you. Based on my research, I believe the very best physical movement is using a mini-trampoline (rebounder). The extremely significant advantage of the rebounder is that you are exercising *every cell* of your body, including your organs, and not just certain muscle groups. This is because of the repetitive acceleration and deceleration of the entire body every time you rebound.

Here's what Henry Savage, M.D. said about the rebounder:

"Never in my 35 years as a practicing physician have I found any exercise method, for any price, that will do more for the physical body than rebound exercise."

"Rebound exercise is the closest thing to the Fountain of Youth that science has found," states James R. White, Ph.D.

According to a study done by NASA – Ames Research Center, published in the <u>Journal of Applied Physiology</u>, *"The external work output at equivalent levels of oxygen uptake were significantly higher while trampolining than running...the greatest difference was about 68 percent."*

I use my rebounder for about 15 minutes a day, keeping my heart rate between 130 and 150 beats per minute (I wear a monitor). In order to keep a high heart rate, I have found that I need to move my arms and elbows in wide circles and lift either my knees toward my chest or my ankles toward my buttocks as I bounce up. Rebounding is an *excellent* and major deposit into your health account.

To get the most out of my time, I either listen to energetic music or pray while I'm jumping. This way I never get bored but I do get very energized and feel like I'm getting younger at the same time. I've found that even just ten to thirty seconds is energizing and very stress reducing!

An excellent book on this type of physical movement is <u>The New Miracles of REBOUND Exercise</u> by Albert Carter.

Stretching is another valuable component of movement and health. Lie on the floor and stretch every muscle in every direction you can think of. I take about one or two minutes to do this every morning and just before I retire at night. Doing this every day is another deposit into your health account.

Another excellent movement method that seems to have an incredible benefit are the "Fountain of Youth" Movements, based on the book, <u>Ancient Secrets of The Fountain of Youth</u>. I've been using these almost daily for nearly two years. They take five to seven minutes to do. They have been taught by Lucy Beale for twelve years in her "How to be Naturally Thin" classes. They are described in the Appendix.

LITTLE WHEELCHAIRS

Have you heard the phrase, "You lose what you don't use"? What would happen with your arm if you kept it in a sling for a year? What would happen if you volunteered to use a wheelchair for a year any time you were not sleeping? Would you get stronger or weaker? You lose what you don't use, right?

But what if the case was made that it would benefit you to live in a wheelchair because it would protect you from injuries, that your muscles would have the needed "support" and cushioning from the harmful effects of stress? Would you be convinced?

Well, what if we did this just for your feet? All your muscles, tendons and ligaments would have "proper support" so that you would be protected by the supposedly harmful stress from the impact when you walk or run. Plus it will be soft and comfortable and will feel like you are walking on air! But most important, your feet will have the maximum protection from injury!

Are you convinced? Millions of people have been, except they aren't called wheelchairs. They are known as athletic or exercise shoes. Of course they don't look like wheelchairs, but they have the same effect. Any device that *restricts movement* of healthy muscles is not good.

A study of 5000 runners discovered that the incident of injury correlated to the price of the shoe. The higher the price of the shoe, the greater the incident of injury!

According to Dr. Phil Maffetone, author of <u>Complementary Sports Medicine and Training For Endurance</u>, the muscles of the feet (particularly the anterior and post anterior tibial) become weak when they are "supported", since they are not being used as much. This causes the feet to deteriorate, which increases problems not only with the feet, but also with the knees, back and hips.

Cushioned shoes do not absorb shock as advertised! What they actually do is prevent the brain from getting the important sensory signals from the feet. As a result, the brain is not able to *adapt* to the shock that is still there, which makes it more damaging than ever to the joints and spine. This even impairs utilization of oxygen from the lungs!

Dr. Maffetone asserts, and I agree, that the best shoes for your feet are the cheapest ones you can find, such as the Wal Mart Silver series under $10. Flat soles are best. Sandals with flat soles are even better, and the very best is to walk barefooted.

When you are home, it is best to be barefoot. That's what I do.

According to the <u>Berkeley Wellness Newsletter</u>, walking on uneven surfaces also strengthens your feet muscles and thus protects you from injuries that occur because your feet muscles are weak.

MOVING STUCK ENERGY

Everything alive operates on energy. The less energy you have, the less life you have. Most of the time though, the problem is not that there is a true lack of energy in your body. The problem is that there is a *blockage* to the flow of that energy that is there, like a beavers dam blocking the flow of water. That blockage is often caused by toxins, stress, imbalances in your life or negative emotions.

Some very effective approaches to removing blocked energy include: chiropractic, acupuncture (traditional and electronic), and applied kinesiology. Kinesiology is the science of movement, particularly of muscles. Having been trained in all three of these areas, my strong preference is applied kinesiology, and particularly Touch For Health, which is the simplified layperson's version. This is an invaluable natural health care system anyone can easily learn and master for the benefit of their family and themselves in a short time. For more information on this extremely valuable resource, call the Touch For Health Association at (800) 466-8342, or go to www.touch4health.com, www.tfh.org or www.kinesiology.net.

A more sophisticated way of moving energy is with an innovative electronic device that uses micro-currents of electricity. This approach uses specific frequencies to support the body's healing and regeneration powers, frequently with dramatic results. Perhaps the most advanced and effective unit is produced by Bio-Therapeutic Computers, Inc. Though this is used primarily in Europe and Asia for beauty enhancement, such as face-lifts, the health and healing benefits can be almost miraculous. I use one myself and believe that "energetic medicine" has an amazing future. For more information on the remarkable health benefits of this device, call Bio-Therapeutic Computers, Inc. at (800) 234-0836 and ask for a free cassette tape and information.

MOVING TOWARD YOUR FUTURE

Another kind of movement that is essential to obtaining vibrant health and longevity is mental. If your thinking and dreaming about the future is stuck or stagnant, it is a sure sign of aging and the development of disease. To be healthy, you need to be mentally on the move. Make sure you are doing something that is challenging, with a vision of where you want to go.

If you are not moving ahead in your mind, it won't be long before you slow down in your body as well.

Why not make sure that YOU are moving through life following your dream, moving toward your vision on a mission?

TRAINS MOVE FAST!

This fourth strategy, based on the Water dynamic, is about movement. Let's build a little further on the train analogy to give you some further insight into how the Water dynamic applies to your health.

Being on the right track (Fire dynamic), well-connected (Earth dynamic) and avoiding the rocks and bullets (Metal dynamic) will do you little good unless you are *moving!*

Think of a mighty rushing river, moving tons of water through a valley. Trains also are engineered to move, and to move fast.

If your train is not moving, it is inevitable that you will be bored. Plus you'll start to rust and deteriorate. Also, even if you are on the right track, if you are just sitting there, you are likely to get run over!

If your train is moving, but very slowly, you're still likely to get bored with it all and get distracted with other things less important than your mission. If you move too slowly, you'll run out of time. Ancient wisdom, using a different metaphor of a race, tells us to "...*run in such a way that you might WIN!*" (II Cor. 9:24).

So just being on the right track (purpose—Fire dynamic), being well-connected (Earth dynamic) to the tracks, other cars and your crew, and avoiding the dangers of rocks (Metal dynamic) is not enough. You need to keep moving!

Miracle Stories

Bill Turner ~ Stomach Cancer

At the age of fifty-nine my world as an active member of my residential construction company came crashing down when I found myself in the hospital with stomach cancer. The tumor was removed, but complications set in and there was a blood clot the entire length of my leg. A filter had to be installed and I found I was allergic to many of the drugs they tried.

A year later a follow-up test found two additional cancerous tumors. The doctors wanted to operate, but I said "no."

The following year more tests found Barrettes esophagus, four ulcers, and an additional tumor. The original tumors had grown. My cholesterol level had risen to 280.

In the fall of 1997 I was introduced to the strategies for vibrant health and longevity. My follow-up test in January 1999 found the Barrettes esophagus reduced in size, the ulcers were gone, and only one tumor remained, but had not grown.

I was feeling very depressed when I couldn't work in our business, and knowing the medical field did not have anything to build me up. The strategies regulated my hormones and lifted my spirits. I was able to pour and finish twelve yards of concrete a few weeks ago.

Carrie Balfanz ~ Pregnancy problems; Urinary Tract Infections

I am a stay-at-home mom with three boys. My first two pregnancies had been miserable. I was extremely sick, vomiting the entire nine months. I had numerous urinary tract infections, was toxemic, anemic, had pre-eclampsia and put on bed rest. There was also the emotional strain of feeling so ill.

Alas, I was introduced to the principles for vibrant health. Low and behold I became pregnant with our third child one year later. Things were definitely different. NO morning sickness, NO swelling, NONE! I had one UTI that disappeared on its own much to my obstetrician's dismay. I rarely needed an afternoon nap and best of all I felt better than ever! Everyone told me, "it must be a girl and so your hormones are just different this time around." "Well, surprise! It's a boy, again!"

Not only was this pregnancy better than the previous two, but this new boy of mine is a much calmer, happier, definitely healthier child. I am living proof that pregnancy can and should be a wonderful experience.

Joan Hearnsberger ~ Epstein-Barr virus, Allergies, Chronic Anemia, Candida & Premenstrual Syndrome

At the ripe old age of twenty-eight, I stared ahead thinking if this is what it would be like to be thirty, I don't think I want to be forty, much less fifty or sixty.

I had a baby and a three year old, and was so tired I could not get up and function before nine or ten in the mornings. After lunch, there were many days that I stationed my little girls in front of the TV while I lay on the sofa nearby half asleep for much of the afternoon. Often my husband would return from work to find that if there was to be any dinner, he would have to cook it.

I had begun to experience joint pain that worsened in the late afternoon to the point that I could not even lift a small sauce pan containing just enough water to heat a small jar of baby food, much less open the jar!

The diagnosis I had at the time was Epstein-Barr virus, allergies, chronic anemia, candida, and a new name for depression and extreme irritability - - premenstrual syndrome.

There were tests for lupus, rheumatoid arthritis, and other autoimmune diseases. Nothing was definitive at the time, but I was told that any of those could eventually become positive. The joint pain, I was told, may have been from a virus, or left over from the bouts of rheumatic fever I was plagued with as a young child.

At this point I begged the Lord to give me guidance. I told Him no matter how weird the answer was I would share anything that helped me with others that had the same problems and no answers. But I continued to suffer while taking shots and other treatments. That was twenty years ago!

In 1996, upon recommendation of a friend, we tried the strategies for vibrant health when my daughter came down with mononucleosis. Two weeks later she went on a ten day whitewater rafting and mountain climbing trip!

Our entire family now uses the strategies. I believe the Lord is restoring the years that the locusts had eaten. My greatest problem now is getting to bed before midnight.

Hildegard Peschel ~ eighty-years-old ~ Excessive weight loss
Before a friend shared the strategies for vibrant health in 1994, I had been losing weight for two and a half years and was unable to find the reason why. Three months after I started, my weight stabilized and I was able to gain enough back to feel good.

Derek & Carol Tozer ~ son with Chronic Eczema

Our first son, Nathaniel, was an extremely colicky, high needs baby, in spite of ecological breastfeeding and attachment parenting. He had his third routine vaccination at seven months of age, and after a few days his skin went from perfectly smooth to a severe case of chronic eczema. We were so shocked we actually took him to the emergency room at our local hospital.

Looking back, it seems obvious that the vaccination caused the eczema. But at the time, we did not make this connection as we were unaware of the risks of vaccination. We tend to think the colic may have been related to candida, but we are not sure.

Nathaniel's eczema and colic were what really led us to begin our desperate search for better health. We tried everything! We started with medical doctors including a dermatologist. Each of them immediately prescribed a drug for our little baby, which we refused. Then we tried helpful chiropractors, and many, many, many health products — but his eczema still persisted. Fortunately, through this experience we learned a great deal about healthy eating. We try to avoid artificial food additives, artificial sweeteners, hydrogenated oil, refined sugar, white flour, caffeine, etc.

A couple of years ago, we were introduced to the strategies for vibrant health by both a chiropractor and a nutritionist. By only trying them a little, we feel we did not give them a chance to work. Earlier this year, as a result of prayer, we tried the strategies consistently. Nathaniel's eczema has completely disappeared! We also notice that he is not as hyper as he used to be, and obeys much quicker. We believe Nathaniel's health improvements are due to the strategies.

Pam McCallister ~ son with Gastroesophageal Reflux Disorder and ear infections; son with Bronchitis and Asthma

My two-year-old son Joel was diagnosed soon after birth with gastroesophageal reflux disorder (GERD) and was on medication. He was supposed to have outgrown it, but at one year old was worse than ever. One complication was frequent ear infections.

After starting Joel on the strategies for vibrant health, he started to show improvement after twenty-four hours. His ears cleared up and have not been a problem since. He has become a happy, healthy child and I am so thankful to the Lord.

My three year old has always been a sick child. His colds always became bronchitis. Antibiotics were our regular routine. Once he got bronchiolitis and from then on he had asthma. I remember the first time I had to rush him to the doctor's office for a breath mist treatment to help him breathe. I was told that the medicine they prescribed could cause esophageal bleeding and hyperactivity. I didn't fill the prescriptions. I went home and tried the strategies for vibrant health.

Six months later he was completely symptom free and could get over a cold in less than a week with no additional infections.

Nordina Newton ~ Eczema, Allergies

My story should start when I was born plagued with skin problems. As I got older I began to develop a lot of allergies that made my life uncomfortable. The straw that broke the camel's back was a recent outbreak of eczema, which covered most of my body. I went to my doctor in desperation feeling like he would wave a magic wand and make it better. Boy was I wrong! My doctor told me he felt that it was "sympathy eczema" due to the fact my hands had been so bad. He sent me to a dermatologist who was very well regarded. I held out hope that the specialist would know what to do. In the next couple of weeks while waiting to see the doctor I got rid of any soap that may have been affecting me, quit washing my clothes in detergents, and waited.

A couple of days later my mother-in-law called me. She wanted me to try the strategies for vibrant health. Now I have no more eczema or allergies, and best of all I have mega energy.

Nancy Kempf ~ Hypoglycemia, Depression

I have had hypoglycemia for approximately twenty-five years. I was told there was little I could do besides eating a special diet, and basically just living with it.

When I began to experience premenopausal symptoms at the age of forty-six, my adrenal glands became depleted. I was in depression most of the time! My energy level and motivation went to an all time low. I spent the next two years lying on the sofa.

One year ago I tried the strategies for vibrant health. Within one week I was experiencing energy that I had never had before! I was able to put in a full day at work and make it through the evening without collapsing. What a great feeling!

Cynde Tilton ~ Asthma

My children and I developed full-blown asthma in the fall of 1996. In the spring I had airtight windows put in, replacing the leaky windows.

The first fall and winter with asthma was very tiring. I not only had to take care of myself, but also care for my two young children. Many nights we required nebulizer-breathing treatments every four hours. I would get three hours sleep, only to get back up and do it all over again. Gradually as spring came the symptoms got better, and we only had to use inhalers four times a day.

The second winter was worse. I had worse asthma requiring steroids, which allowed me to breathe while having horrible side effects. I couldn't believe this was how I would have to live the rest of my life. I was so depressed and sick and tired of being sick and tired.

My family started using the strategies for vibrant health in July, and in two months my daughter was off her inhalers. She hasn't had any asthma flare-ups since. My son and I had an incredibly easy winter. We still had colds, but the asthma wasn't as bad.

Jane Emanuel ~ Arthritis

I first began experiencing arthritic pain about fifteen years ago. Over the years the pain gradually worsened, until I was in extreme pain, mostly in my feet, hips, and hands. I could no longer open a jar or soft drink can. I could barely write or drive my car. I could no longer saddle up my horse, much less ride without pain. And as a horse massage therapist, I couldn't even think about massaging a horse.

I was on a search for a natural product that would help me, since I don't like taking drugs unless absolutely necessary. (I was taking

*aspirin to help control the pain.) I tried many natural products over
the years, none of which helped at all. But I still knew that there had
to be something out there that could help me. I just needed to find it.*

*In my search, I contacted a friend who steered me in the direction of
some new health strategy. I decided to give it a try. By the end of six
weeks my pain was gone. I realized that I was no longer making regular trips to the aspirin bottle, and then realized I wasn't experiencing
any pain. I was pretty amazed.*

*How has this changed my life? I am back to saddling up my horse
and I can ride for several hours without pain. I'm back to massaging
horses, and I can do everything I did before I experienced pain. This
has been a true blessing for me. I will continue to do what I need to do
to stay healthy.*

Norman R. Piersma ~ Metastatic Melanoma

*"You have, maximum, six months to live," said my oncologist eight
years ago. Having seen three other patients of his die within five
months of metastatic melanoma, I knew he was telling the truth. So I
said, "no" to his proposed chemo treatments. We prayed to the Lord
for guidance and started looking for answers.*

*After weeks of natural therapy and new orientation in Mexico, we
began a whole new life based on the principles of WELLNESS. I've
done well. I am now the Florida State Champion in the 5K race walk
among men aged seventy to seventy-four. But in spite of all the grace
of God and victory of these years, my intense search for the best therapy
was getting confusing. One year ago a friend told me about the
strategies for vibrant health. Our quest was over - - these strategies
were our answer.*

Crystal Porter ~ Ovarian Carcinoma

*To give the details of my ordeal would take months. Instead, let me
simply say that I was told by my doctor that I had ovarian carcino-
ma, stage three to four. One tumor grew through my colon causing a
blockage. The surgeon removed the tumors and repaired the colon. The
surgery weakened my colon and it burst a few days later. Soon peri-*

*tonitis spread through my abdomen. The doctor later told me they did-
n't think I'd live another couple months.*

*I had another surgery and was given a temporary colostomy, and
started chemotherapy. I was very sick and lost about forty pounds.*

*In June of 1996 I went into surgery to have my colostomy reversed
and the surgeon found a hole in my colon, called a fistula. He
repaired that and sent me home for six weeks to recover. By August,
I was strong enough to have my colostomy reversed. The incision
had healed leaving a two inch wide scar, which was reopened and
removed. The doctor also explored the pelvic area, removing scar
tissue, lymph nodes, and giving me a biopsy. I soon learned that
the tissue, lymph nodes, and rinse were all concentrated with
thousands of small tumors. My oncologist suggested an experimental
chemotherapy called Topotican. She gave me a 17 percent chance
of recovery.*

*In November of 1996, after trying Topotican for four months, I
quit taking the chemotherapy. Soon a tumor showed up growing on my
pelvic muscle. The doctor was surprised because only one small tumor
was detected instead of thousands. It was so small that my doctor
suggested we wait before trying surgery. It was in a bad spot among
nerves to my legs and the chances were high for paralysis.*

*In July of 1997 I tried the strategies for vibrant health. Not only
did my tumor growth slow way down, but also my memory and
clarity of mind were almost immediately recovered. My strength and
stamina began to return. My neuropathy recovered about 70 percent
and I did not catch one infection.*

*Although I had another bout with cancer (this time ovarian cancer),
I continued with the strategies. My husband and I agreed to try the
chemo again, as well, but it didn't help. When my doctor wanted me to
do the chemo again, I refused. So she suggested another CAT scan to see
what the tumor was doing.*

*On August 15, 1998 I received a phone call from the doctor. The
tumor had disintegrated and started to calcify (die)! The scan showed
there was no visible activity.*

*Here it is 1999 and it has been a year since my last chemotherapy.
My tumor counts are getting high again, and the doctor started me on
carboplatnum chemotherapy. I have had four treatments and have two*

more to go. I have been sicker this time than in the past months. I believe this is because I haven't been using the strategies to health.

Brenda L. Renrick ~ Back Pain, Arthritis, Skin, Eyes, Stress, PMS, Asthma, Allergies

I started using some of the principles of vibrant health on October 8, 1995, after a friend had shared some of these principles with me. Since that time I have noticed many positive changes. To date they are as follows:

For years I had severe lower back pain and visited the chiropractor frequently. Presently, I have very little back pain. My arthritic knees hurt when I walked and exercised. Now my knees feel wonderful after exercising. Exercise has truly been a more pleasant experience since I know I will not be in pain.

I am also losing weight since learning how to eat based on my body's profile.

My skin is much smoother and softer. In the past I have had a series of facial outbreaks and lichen planus. Lichen planus is an unpleasant skin disease that surfaces on various parts of the body skin in a tree-like format. Now I have none of these skin problems.

My eyes were examined December 18, 1995, and my vision had improved by fifty percent. In May of 1996, my eyes were examined again and they had improved fifteen percent more. Now, I wear only one contact lens for reading. When I am not wearing the contact, I use a pair of "reading" glasses.

My doctor had prescribed the drug Buspar to relieve stress and anxiety. Now, I've stopped taking Buspar. I have much more energy, am more focused, have very little stress, and I sleep more soundly during the night.

I also experienced some positive hormonal changes that have served to correct a problem I have had since puberty. My "monthly challenges" are much easier, and I am noticeably less irritable.

Another added benefit is my hair grows much faster, the natural color is much more dominant than ever before. I also have great fingernails.

Lastly, I use very little of my asthma and no allergy medicines. I had taken allergy injections for twenty-one years (over 250 monthly injections). I have not had an injection since October '96.

Since I abused my body for so many years with drugs, alcohol and tobacco, I know my story is just beginning to unfold. Thank God for these principles of health!!!!

Dave, Shirley, Joseph (8) and Sarah (6.5) Williams Family with an autistic child; Insulin Reduction

We live in a small town in Alberta, Canada called Barrhead. Dave is a juvenile diabetic, I (Shirley) have weight problems, and our son, Joseph, is mildly autistic but high functioning. We have experimented with the strategies for vibrant health for Joseph for the past two years.

Some of the problems Joseph was having are as follows: tantrums, talking to himself, reciting videos over and over, numerous food allergies, and asthma. He also experienced speech and language delays, short attention span, poor social behaviors, and inability to pretend or use his imagination, and low energy are just some of the symptoms Joseph exhibited.

Upon trying the strategies for vibrant health, we have noticed significant improvements including: less tantrums, lengthened attention span, more conversation, improved speech and language, allergies are less severe. He also catches fewer colds and seems to have a longer attention span.

My husband, Dave, has reduced his insulin intake by 30 percent and can go longer between meals without getting low blood sugar levels.

I have had a life-long battle with weight and female problems. Since I have been using the strategies for vibrant health I have had better weight maintenance and less problems with premenstrual syndrome.

Overall, our whole family is much stronger, has more energy, endurance, and resilience.

7

NOURISHING YOUR HEALTH
(The Wood Dynamic)

Nourishment

Quality

Quality Control

Altered Food

When Fat Becomes Ugly

Quantity

Ratios are Vital

The Big FAT Lie

Two Hidden Dangers of Losing Weight

Variety is Vital

Fanatic or Passionate?

Leader of the Pack
The Essential Nutrients
The Good, Bad and the Ugly
Fighting Fat with Fat
Super Sugars
Health Insurance You Can Eat
Dr. See's Landmark Study
What is Your Real Age?
Trains Need Fuel!
Miracle Stories

NOURISHMENT

The fifth and final strategy to your health and longevity is in the Wood dynamic. Wood is a symbol of growth and nourishment. Living in the northwest, I picture a tall majestic Douglas fir. With the proper conditions, these trees can grow for centuries. In this book, wood is going to represent nourishment and nutrition, the source of which is food, and food alone.

It is often in this fifth strategy that people experience the fastest and most dramatic results in health recovery and freedom. People have frequently reported noticeable and sometimes dramatic improvement within the first 24 hours. Sometimes it will be in several days, weeks or even six months before the big breakthrough happens. What is going to make the biggest difference is giving your body or mind that which is most severely deficient, such as missing essential nutrients.

There are five critical elements regarding food that are extremely vital to vibrant health and longevity. They are *quality, quantity, ratios* of the three basic groups, *variety*, and *essential nutrients*. Just as all five of the strategies are important to having vibrant health and longevity, all five of these elements are extremely important to your health as well. Neglecting them is the same as writing "stress checks." You can't afford to leave even one out if you are sincerely committed to vibrant health, happiness and longevity.

QUALITY

Ever heard the phrase, "garbage in—garbage out"? Or "you reap according to how you sow"? Your body is no exception. What would happen to your car if you put in poor quality fuel? The same thing happens when we feed ourselves poor quality food. *As a nation, we are overfed and under-nourished.*

Let's establish this up front. I say you *deserve* the highest quality food there is, because you are important and the quality of your life is important. Do you agree? There is too much at stake (i.e. your life!) to do anything less than give yourself the best. Doesn't it make sense that if you settle for *poor quality food*, such as junk food, that eventually you will have to settle for a *poor quality life?* Do you really want to pay the price for that costly mistake and be a statistic in the health disaster, as will 95 percent of Americans?

Would you build your house out of junk lumber and cheap materials, even if it were more convenient and less expensive at the time?

Many people would not be caught dead driving a junk car, but are unaware (or live in denial) that they *will* be literally caught dead in a "junk body" when their health "accident" occurs.

If you need to eat something fast and convenient, most types of Mexican fast food are not too bad. My first choice is to eat a nutrient dense protein bar that is uniquely based on whole food technology, and is a nutrient delivery system for what many researchers and doctors believe to be the top three nutraceutical/nutritional complexes in the world. For me, they are the ultimate in quality, taste and convenience.

The issue is not always junk food. Sometimes the choice is between good, better and best. For example, iceberg lettuce is not considered junk food. Although it is natural and unprocessed, it is void of many of the nutrients found in other types of lettuce. Boston or Bibb lettuce has twice as much Vitamin C and three times as much beta carotene by weight as iceberg lettuce. Even better, Romaine has six times as much Vitamin C and eight times as much beta-carotene and far more chlorophyll than iceberg. Alfalfa sprouts are even more nutritious.

QUALITY CONTROL

There are *three factors* that determine the quality of your food. The first critical factor is one that is the hardest to do anything about: the quality of the soil in which it is grown. Because most soil is depleted by 80 to 90 percent of many of the essential minerals we need for healthy bodies, the plants that we eat also lack many of the minerals and nutrients we need.

For example, there is a direct correlation between the levels of remaining selenium in soil and the rate of cancer in that area—the lower the selenium levels, the greater the incidence of cancer.

In addition, the toxic cancer-causing pesticides added to the nutrient-deficient foods (hidden "stress checks") add even more stress to your body.

Processing the Life Out of *Your Food*

The second factor that determines the quality of your food is commercial *processing*. Most foods start off as good and natural, but are easily ruined by processing that occurs *before* they are consumed. Much of the processed food we consume, especially wheat, rice and corn (the ultimate processed, nutrient- deficient food is white sugar), have been seriously altered by having most of their vital nutrients stripped away so that the "food" can be stored longer. Processed foods do not spoil as fast.

Then the processors have the nerve to deceptively label this incomplete nutrient-stripped food as "enriched" or "fortified" by adding back a few inorganic minerals (from ground up rocks) and synthetic vitamins (mostly from petroleum). How much do you think this compensates for the many naturally occurring nutrients that had been removed?

It's like a thief that is stealing 90 percent of your pay check every month and claiming he is enriching you by giving you a $20 bonus.

It only "enriches" the pockets of the processors (nutrient thieves), while further robbing your body of essential minerals and nutrients.

The worst victims of this deception are the children. They get ripped off and hurt the worst because they trust their parents, who believe the advertisers. I find it absolutely astounding that "Wonder Bread" was allowed for years to promote the lie that their bread built strong bodies 12 ways. The Federal Trade Commission *finally* made them stop advertising that claim (lie).

Processing for Life

The processing that is actually very important for your health is the processing that is supposed to happen *after* the food is in your mouth. This processing is done by chewing your food until it becomes liquified.

This is further enhanced by having a heartfelt appreciation for your food (a huge deposit into your health account). Many people do this through a heart felt prayer of gratitude. Get even greater value by enjoying your meal in a relaxed state of mind, which includes sitting down. Eating while standing up tenses numerous muscles, and interferes with digestion. Especially do not eat when you are stressed or upset for the same reason.

The second stage of internal processing (digestion) is done by the hydrochloric acid in your stomach. Most people over forty produce insufficient amounts of hydrochloric acid (HCL), and often times none, when they are under stress. If you are over forty, you would do well to consider taking HCL as a digestive aid. Ignore the ads that want you to believe that you are producing too much acid. It is far more likely that you are producing far too little, especially if you are under a lot of stress.

It is also better not to dilute the hydrochloric acid you do have by drinking a lot of liquid during your meals. Consider supporting the final stage of digestion by using a high quality enzyme supplement.

Any food that is not fully digested is stressful to your body and becomes toxic, and therefore, another "stress check" to your health account.

Additives that Subtract

The third factor that determines the quality of your food is the additives and preservatives added into most processed foods. Also the antibiotics fed to animals is another serious health threat to those who eat that meat. All these chemicals create more stress and work for your body, further depleting your precious reserves and lowering the balance in your health account.

ALTERED FOOD

Because nutrient-stripped foods, such as refined sugar, bleached flour and white rice have been *altered*, they are imbalanced, like having a flat tire on your car. Imbalanced foods are very stressful to your body. As serious "stress checks," they can create serious chemical and energy imbalances within your body, which is the last thing you need!

Another example of an altered food is dairy products. Milk is inherently a great wholesome food, *until it is altered*. Then it becomes a "stress check."

These are my four concerns:

1. **Pasteurization** alters 42 percent of the proteins, which prevent them from being assimilated. If a farmer feeds a calf with pasteurized milk, it dies. The famous Price-Pottinger cat study tracked the effects of pasteurized milk and cooked meat over four generations. By the second generation, the bones and organs deteriorated and the cats lost their hair. The third generation started showing homosexual tendencies. The fourth generation was sterile. Right now we're about three generations into using pasteurization.
2. **Homogenization**, another way milk is altered, is a cause of heart disease according to Dr. William Ellis, a retired

osteopathic physician and surgeon, and past president of the American Academy of Applied Osteopathy. There is an enzyme in cow's milk called Xanthine Oxidase (XO) that attacks the heart's arteries. In unhomogenized (unaltered) milk, this is not a problem because our bodies can break down the XO and excrete it. But the homogenization process reduces the fat globules in milk to such a tiny size (which is why the cream does not rise to the top) that the XO can not be excreted, and is instead absorbed into the blood stream. From there it attacks the heart and artery tissues. Then the body patches up the damage with cholesterol.

Dr. Kurt Esselbacher, the past chairman of the Department of Medicine of the Harvard Medical School states, *"Homogenized milk, because of its XO content, is one of the major causes of heart disease in the U.S."*

Research done by Dr. Kurt A. Oster, Chief of Cardiology at Park City Hospital, Bridgeport, Connecticut, reported this from a study of 75 patients with angina pectoris and atherosclerosis: *"All the patients were taken off milk and given folic acid and vitamin C, both of which combat the action of XO. The results were dramatic. Chest pains decreased, symptoms lessened and each one of those patients is doing great today."*

3. **Growth hormones and antibiotics** given to cows to stimulate increased milk production pass through to the milk. This has been shown to have a negative impact on human health. In fact, a British Medical Journal study on the loss of libido in men attributed it to the poultry industry feeding chickens female hormones to speed up their growth. As a result, men were getting an increased bust.

4. **Allergies** are a serious problem. It is estimated that as much as 90 percent of the American population is allergic to milk, which makes it a "stress check" just on this basis.

According to the Journal of the American Medical Association

(Nov. 1997), food allergies are the number one cause of recurrent ear infections in children, and milk is the biggest culprit. Eliminating milk would stop infections in nearly 50 percent of kids. Eliminating sugar, pop and juices from their diets would prevent 50-70 percent of the remaining infections.

There are excellent alternatives, such as raw milk if available (raw goats milk is best for children), soy milk, almond milk, rice milk, and of course the best beverage is pure water. Unless you are allergic to soy, the best substitute is probably soy milk, which is what I use.

If you are an open-minded person, I urge you to visit www.notmilk.com or www.antidairycoalition.com to see the research and documentation on the serious problems and misinformation on dairy products.

WHEN FAT BECOMES UGLY

Another food that is *altered* is oil, either by hydrogenation or simply by heating it. In either case, it becomes what is called **trans fat**. A study in the New England Journal of Medicine (Nov. 1997) showed that whereas saturated fat (from meat and dairy) increased heart disease risk by 17 percent, *trans fat increased it by 93 percent.*

Although French fries, potato and corn chips or any fried foods taste great in your mouth, they are like a Trojan horse or a time bomb in your body! Any time oil is heated, dangerous free radicals are produced that not only accelerate the aging and disease process, but put a heavy burden on your immune system. Do you want these kinds of "stress checks" against your health account?

Using foods with trans oil (heated oil or partially hydrogenated) is like *sabotaging* your own immune system. It is like poking holes in your boat out on the ocean because it seems fun at the time! It won't be fun, however, when you start to sink!

If you must use oil for cooking, use butter or organic coconut oil because they are already completely saturated and no trans fat can be made from them. Extra virgin olive oil (not "pure" or light) is next best for cooking and definitely best for overall use. It's better to add some unheated oil (cold pressed and unrefined) or butter to your food *after* it is cooked. According to Dr. Mary Enig (internationally renowned trans fat investigator), it is best to totally avoid using Canola (rapeseed), corn or soy oil.

For a shocking eye opening education on trans fat, go to the web and search for hydrogenated oil.

Perhaps the most insidious type of food alteration, and predicted by some to be the most disastrous in the long term, is the genetic engineering of foods which has been banned by many countries.

It's Your Choice

While our cells and bodies are screaming bloody murder, our uninformed taste buds are dancing with delight and begging for more! Is it any surprise that 95 percent of us die from heart/vascular disease, cancer and diabetes?

What can you do? You can either live "not knowing" (too late for that now!), pretend that things are not really that bad (denial), or you can make more intelligent choices to reduce the stress and negative impact on your health by the problems just described. You can choose to buy whole food without additives and preservatives, and meat without antibiotics. It will cost you a little more now, and may not be as convenient, but aren't you worth it? *Remember what's at stake—your vibrant health and longevity!*

Decide what you are committed to—your taste buds and convenience, or to life. This is a life or death decision!

At the same time, if you are making intelligent healthy choices

95 percent of the time (a lot of deposits to your health account), your body will most likely be able to handle the other 5 percent of less than ideal choices ("stress checks"). I still eat refined and altered foods, such as sugar and refined white flour, altered dairy products, such as ice cream, but only *occasionally*—I just don't do it every day! I value my health too much! My body can handle this stuff once or twice a month as long as I'm eating intelligently with integrity 95 percent of the time.

However, if you are facing a serious health challenge (your health account is experiencing "bounced checks"), you may not have the luxury of being any less than 100 percent compliant with making the best choices.

QUANTITY

The second critical element that is vital to your vibrant health and longevity is the *quantity* of food you eat. If you were to go on a long hike, perhaps up a mountain, isn't it true that the more weight you carried, the less distance you could go? The same is true of eating food—the more we eat, the less years we live. Aging slows down in monkeys who eat a well-balanced diet with the calorie content reduced by 30 percent, according to a published study by Dr. George Roth, a scientist at the gerontology research center of the National Institute on Aging, part of the National Institutes of Health.

"We (science) have known for 70 years that if you fed mice less food, they age slower, live longer and get diseases less frequently," he said.

More Eating Equals Less Living!

According to Dr. Barbara Hansen, half of the monkeys on unrestricted diets (sounds like most of us) died prematurely (sounds like the 95 percent), while only 12.5 percent of those on calorie-restricted diets died at an early age! Plus, restricting calories reduced the rate of cancer, heart disease and diabetes in the test animals (aren't these the top three causes of death in humans? Interesting!).

Dr. Thomas Perls, director of the New England Centenarian Study and co-author of the book, *Living to 100*, found that almost 100 percent of people who live more than 100 years had eaten in moderation. Ancient wisdom from the Bible tells us the same thing: do all things in moderation.

Be a Centenarian!

If you want to be a healthy centenarian (living past age 100), and I challenge you to seriously make that one of your health goals, moderation is a critical strategy that you cannot afford to ignore. Overeating (a serious "stress check") is a slow but sure way to premature disease and death, which is a huge price to pay in exchange for some short term taste bud pleasure in your mouth.

Another critical factor that supports longevity in a major way is choosing and consuming a diet of primarily low glycemic index foods. More about that later.

One of the ways to overcome the almost universal compulsion to overeat is to use a simple technique taught by Lucy Beale in her excellent tape album, "How to be a Naturally Thin Person." All you need to do is eat *only* when you are hungry (NEVER eat when you are upset), and then only eat until you reach a five on a scale from zero to ten. Ten is uncomfortably stuffed—I'm sure you know the feeling! Zero is a definite discomfort in your stomach. Five is when you've eaten enough to remove the discomfort. There are many other excellent tips to normalizing your weight in this album.

You Need a Break - Take the Whole Day Off!

Another thing to consider doing is to fast one day a week - abstain from food. Not only does this give your digestive system a much needed break, but it stops any momentum you may have been building up from overeating. My wife and I do this every week, usually on Wednesdays, and I find it to be extremely helpful in terms of breaking the cycle of eating too much, which is so easy for me to do. I really enjoy the benefits I get from fasting one day a week. It is a great deposit into my health account. Also there is some great spiritual value in doing this if you want to do it for that reason as well.

If you have a blood sugar problem or tire easily, you may want to do a partial fast, and have vegetable (not fruit) juices or a whole food protein bar. If it is too difficult to do a whole day, begin by just skipping dinner. That's how I started.

Another time to abstain from food is when you are not feeling well or you are stressed out. Animals do this instinctively. By not eating when you are sick, the energy that would be used for digestion can now be used for the healing process, so you can recover faster. However, double your intake of water!

If you eat when you are upset, your digestive system does not work well, and the partially digested food ends up being toxic to your system (another "stress check").

The later that you eat during the day, the more the food will be stored as fat. Ideally, it is best to have your last meal by five or six o'clock, and avoid evening or late night snacks. If you get hungry, drink some water, and perhaps a fiber supplement with it.

RATIOS ARE VITAL

The third critical element in the nutrition arena is eating the proper *ratios* of protein, carbohydrates (a long complex chain of sugar molecules) and fats at each meal. The ratio of foods can often be more important than the kind of food you eat. This is based on the fact that "one shoe does not fit all." Many people, because of their ancestry and genetics, absolutely need higher ratios of protein (40 to 45 percent) and fat (10 to 20 percent) in their diet, and will become sick if they consume too high a percentage of carbohydrates. This is especially typical of people of

European descent, but not always.

Even good food in the wrong ratio is a "stress check" against your account.

Did you realize that as much as 70 percent of the carbohydrates you eat can be turned into fat by your own body? This is even worse if they are eaten at night.

To avoid this unpleasant surprise, eat some protein with each meal and keep the carbohydrates down to 30 to 40 percent of the meal. In fact, *any* food, including salads, fruit and meat, will be turned to fat if you overeat.

On the other hand, some people absolutely need higher ratios of carbohydrates (50 to 70 percent) in their diet, and do not do well if they consume too high a percentage of protein and fat. These people do well as vegetarians. This is especially typical of people of Eastern Indian descent, but not always.

Whether you are a fast or slow oxidizer is a reflection of your metabolic rate and is referred to as metabolic profiling. You will fit into one of three basic profiles. These will tell you which of three ratios is best to give you the most energy and vibrant health.

Your Body Knows Best by Ann Louise Gittleman is an excellent book on this subject. The book includes a free profiling test that will show you in 15 minutes which metabolic profile type you are. Implementing this important information can make an immediate and major difference in your energy levels and health.

THE BIG FAT LIE

Over two thirds of Americans are over weight, and half of them are considered obese. Most of the remaining third of Americans are concerned about becoming overweight! While we are obsessed with avoiding food that is high in fat, America has the dubious distinction of its population having the highest percentage of overweight people of any nation in the world! England is number two!

One of the most common and harmful misunderstandings is the misinformation (lie) that we are fat because we eat too much fat.

Though eating excess fat can contribute, the primary culprit for excess body fat and many degenerative diseases such as heart disease, cancer and diabetes is NOT eating foods high in fat, but eating too much carbohydrates and sugar, and especially in combination with fat, such as french fries and corn or potato chips. People on a high carbohydrate and low fat diet tend to be more unhealthy, carry more excess body fat, and don't live as long.

Putting the Brakes to Your Metabolism!

What creates excess body fat, more than anything else, is a high RATIO of the carbohydrates to protein and fat, and especially certain *types* of carbohydrates that have a *high conversion rate to fat*. When the percentage of a *meal* (not just for the day) is higher in sugar or carbohydrates (a long chain of sugar molecules), much more of that food will be converted to fat instead of being burned as energy (calories). The effect of this is *putting the brakes on your metabolism*, which results in lower energy and greater storage of fat. Obviously, this is NOT what you want!

Plus this sets up a vicious cycle of overeating. Once the carbohydrates are converted to fat, you get a blood sugar drop, which makes you hungry for more carbohydrates. So you eat more to raise your blood sugar, and the whole vicious cycle repeats! Soon, you've gained weight, and feel even more like a failure.

According to the Glycemic Research Institute, many of the "fat-free" foods are much more fattening than they were before the fat was removed, because sugar has been added (and often disguised) to compensate for the low fat!

This is because carbohydrates and sugar, and especially certain carbohydrates, stimulate insulin production. Insulin directs your body to convert the food to fat and store it as fat instead of just burning it as energy. To measure this fat conversion and storage effect, foods are rated by what is called the glycemic index. *The higher the index, the higher percentage of that food <u>and the other foods eaten with it</u>, will be converted to fat, regardless of the fat content of the food.*

So for an example, eating high glycemic foods like baked potato, corn flakes or cooked oatmeal which are low in fat, is more fattening than eating a juicy beef steak or a bowl of ice cream!

High Fat Conversion Foods

These are some common foods with their glycemic index numbers, that are especially *high* on this index, and thus stimulate fat storage:

Common sugar (sucrose)—92
Macaroni and cheese—92
Potatoes (mashed—100; French fries—107; baked—121; potato chips—high)
Corn—78; pop corn—79; corn chips—105; corn flakes—119
Pizza—86
White rice—83; brown rice—79
White and wheat bread—101
Cold cereals (most). E.g. Life—94; Grapenuts—96; Cheerios—106; Total—109
Cooked cereals (e.g. Cream of Wheat—100, oatmeal—87 (steel cut is less)
Bananas—77
Carrots—70
Most juices and all drink mixes and soft drinks (97)
Desserts (ice cream—87); donuts—108
Fat-free bottled "lite" dressings (due to added corn syrup and maltodextrins).
High fructose corn syrup—89
Maltodextrins—150 (added to many foods, but deceptively not counted as sugar!)

Did you notice that some of these foods are worse than pure sugar? It is wise to eat these foods sparingly. And when you do eat these foods, balance the glycemic index for the whole meal by eating low index foods with them.

Fat Burning Foods

Here are some of the foods that are rated as having a *low* glycemic index:

Fructose—32
Trutina Dulcem (a fruit sugar fifteen times sweeter
than regular sugar)
"Super sugars" (glyconutrients)
Stevia—though not "approved" by the FDA as a
sweetener, it is often used as such
High protein foods (e.g. fish, meat and eggs)
Most vegetables including *sweet* potatoes and yams
Beans—40
Salads—low
Avocado—low
Stone ground bread and sprouted grain—low
Barley—36
Rye—48
Most pastas—varies; spaghetti—59 (but very low
nutritional value)
Berries—low
Cherries—32
Apples—54
Oranges—63
Peaches—60
Pears—53
Dairy products; whole milk—39 (there are other
concerns mentioned previously)
Soy milk—43
Seeds and nuts—as low as 21 (peanuts)

Butter (in moderation—far superior to margarine)
Olive oil
Soy beans—25
Celery—very very low

There is another huge advantage to using low glycemic foods besides weight control: *longevity!* According to a study by T. Par entitled "Insulin Exposure and Aging Theory" in the *Journal Gerontology* - 1997; 43:182-200, high insulin levels, which result from consuming high glycemic foods, *promote accelerated aging.*

Both calorie restriction and a low glycemic index diet appear to be important for longevity, BUT a diet of low glycemic foods is even more effective than calorie restriction for longevity.

For more information on glycemic indexing of foods, visit the web site of the Glycemic Research Institute at www.glycemic.com and www.mendosa.com/gilists.htm.

TWO HIDDEN DANGERS OF LOSING WEIGHT

Most people who lose weight are *less* healthy as a result of it. One reason is because most weight loss is primarily the result of losing fluids and lean muscle tissue, which includes your heart muscle and other vital organs. Almost 100 percent of the time the weight comes back, but whereas the fluid loss is regained, the loss in muscle tissue is not. Instead, it is replaced by fat. The end result is that you are NOT back where you started, though you may think so by looking at the scale; instead, your body composition is altered so that you are now at a higher percentage of fat and your muscle mass is lower. This in turn *decreases* your metabolic rate (the process of turning food into energy vs. storing it as fat), which means that now even more food is stored as fat instead of being burned for energy.

The Center for Science in the Public Interest distributed a news release in June of 1996 entitled, *"Weight-Loss Firms Keep Consumers in the Dark about Prices, Effectiveness. Health Groups Demand FTC Action."* Their report presented highly critical evaluations of the five largest centers: Jenny Craig, Nutri/System, Physicians Weight Loss Centers, Diet Center and Weight Watchers, stating that they *"...fail to tell their potential customers about the full costs of their services, and fail to provide information about how well—or how poorly—they work...."* The biggest failure of the weight loss industry is the distorted focus on weight loss, which is NOT the real issue (except from a marketing perspective).

The real issue is this: the body composition (muscle mass to fat ratio). Losing weight is a false standard and unhealthy illusion. The proper goal is to alter the body composition (less body fat and increased muscle mass) and doing it in such a way that you don't gain it back.

Therefore it is extremely important to make sure that your weight loss is based on losing fat as measured by inches, and not on the false and unreliable standard of losing weight as measured by pounds. One of the most effective ways of doing this is to include in your weight loss strategy a supplement designed to increase both your metabolism rate and your lean muscle mass, along with lifestyle changes such as eating low glycemic index foods and adequate activity. *Otherwise, you may be losing weight temporarily, and losing some of your health permanently!*

What Else Have You Got to Lose?

The second hidden danger of losing weight is that you are likely to be losing still another critical component of health: **bone mineral density** (BMD). This obviously increases the risk of osteoporosis which affects a huge portion of the population. In fact, fifty percent of women over fifty will break a bone; 40 percent of the women with hip fractures never recover, half of them dying within 12 months from complications and the other half ending up in a nursing home unable to care for themselves.

The loss of bone mineral density (BMD) associated with weight loss is based on a recent study reported in the American Journal of Clinical Nutrition, supported in part by the National Institute on Aging, the University of California at San Francisco and the University of Pittsburgh, Graduate School of Public Health. In this clinical trial, 236 healthy premenopausal women aged 44-50 were randomly assigned to intervention and control groups. BMD was measured by Dual Energy X-ray Absorptiometry (a FDA approved technology for measuring bone density) at the lumbar spine and hips before and after 18 months. Dietary fat intake was lowered and physical activity was increased to produce a modest weight loss. Those who did lose weight (not necessarily fat) *lost twice as much BMD at the hip and lumbar spine than did the control group that did not lose weight!*

Even more alarming was that the top 25 percent of the weight losers lost three times as much BMD as the control group who lost no weight!

In a study with a more encouraging outcome, done by Gilbert Kaats, Ph.D. of the Health and Medical Research Foundation in San Antonio Texas, it was discovered that participants in a clinical trial who lost weight *while taking glyconutrients, actually increased BMD by an average of 1.13 percent over a 75 day period.* The norm in the US general population is to lose .25 percent BMD for the same period of time (or 1 percent per year).

<u>VARIETY IS VITAL</u>

The fourth critical element in the nutrition arena is eating a larger *variety* of foods. Most people seem to get stuck in a rut of eating only a very few different kinds of foods.

In fact, people often become allergic to the foods they eat every day, even if it is a good food! A lack of variety is a "stress check" to your account.

Why not broaden your horizons? Why be narrow or limited? Be adventurous! Try new vegetables and different fruits. Try tofu and soy milk, or rice or almond milk. Use grains, like millet, barley, oats, kamut, spelt, etc. Eat raw seeds and nuts every day, such as sunflower and pumpkin seeds, almonds, pecans, macadamia, pistachio or hazelnuts to get some of the essential fats.

Another reason that variety is important to your health is because different foods have different *ratios of nutrients.*

Often, the *ratio* of certain nutrients are more important than the amounts, such as calcium and magnesium, or copper and zinc. Therefore, foods that are almost identical in the basic composition, can have dramatically different impacts on your health and how you feel.

Anti-Terrorists

Furthermore, variety is important because the antioxidant or anti-carcinogenic properties vary dramatically in foods that appear to be pretty much the same. Antioxidants are extremely important deposits to make into your health account because they are like anti-terrorists that neutralize free radicals (internal terrorists), which cause the kind of cellular damage that can lead to cancer, heart disease, arthritis, and even aging. Free radicals, like toxins, damage or mutate cells and disrupt cell to cell communication, which interferes with proper immune system function.

The McDonald's Hamburger Experiment

Here's an example of what the immediate measurable effect of antioxidants can be as reported in a recent <u>Journal of the American Medical Association</u>. Twenty subjects who ate the fat-packed McDonald's breakfast had impaired blood vessel function for up to four hours afterwards. But no such impairment was found on another day when they swallowed 20 times the recommended dosage of certain antioxidants before eating the same meal. But notice it took 20 times the recommended amounts for this effect!

Don't you think you have enough stress that you *can't* avoid? Why add this kind of biochemical assault to your heart and immune system by abusing your self with junk food?

DON'T let your taste buds ruin your health and life! You are the master—don't be a slave to your taste buds. You can't afford the consequences!

FANATIC OR PASSIONATE?

At this point, you may be thinking, "Yeah, but I can't get fanatical about all this health stuff!"

I say, why not? Aren't you "fanatic" about protecting your life when you do whatever it takes to stay on your side of the traffic line when there is oncoming traffic?

Aren't you "fanatic" about protecting the lives of your family members from any kind of danger?

Consider this comparison: The average American adult spends (wastes?) four hours a day (28 hours a week) sitting in front of the TV with no benefit other than a little shallow entertainment. To me *that* sounds fanatic!

It's good to be "fanatic" about something—just make sure it's worthwhile. Why not be "fanatic" (a better word is "passionate") about enhancing and protecting your health (physically, emotionally and spiritually)? Which is worse? To risk the possibility of being thought of as a "fanatic" in regards to your health or to die as part of the 95 percent group? Is following the truth and doing what is best for yourself and family really fanatical or is it just good common sense?

Natural food was the ONLY kind of food for humanity until the 1920's and 30's. To create bigger profits, the food industry stepped up its processing and packaging of foods. It appears that now the pendulum is slowly beginning to swing back to natural foods.

According to Dr. Phil Maffetone, a Sports Nutritional Doctor,

"It's up to each of us to rebel against the trillion-dollar processed-food industry by avoiding junk, choosing only convenience foods made from real food and making our own meals from real ingredients rather than throwing a box of powder in the microwave."

Avoid the S.A.D. or B.A.D.

You don't have to participate in **S.A.D.**—the "**S**tandard **A**merican **D**iet" (also known as **B.A.D.**—the **B**asic **A**merican **D**iet). If you do, it is inevitable that you will someday have some real SAD/BAD news when you find yourself paying the awful price of being in the 95 percent category. You don't have to be a part of the "Sorry Majority."

I saw an interesting cartoon of an Oriental father standing over his son who was sitting on the floor complaining about having to eat his bowl of rice that he held in his hands. The father is saying, *"Eat your rice, son—think of the millions of Americans who have nothing to eat except junk food."*

People usually highly respect those who have the courage to take a stand for a principle that the majority are unwilling to follow. Why not be that kind of person? Why not be different? Why not be smarter? Why not live longer? Why not be in the surviving 5 percent? Not only will you look good, but you'll look and feel good longer!

LEADER OF THE PACK

The U.S. Department of Agriculture's Center for Aging at Tuft's University recently studied more than 40 fruits and vegetables. They discovered that blueberries contained the highest level of antioxidants of all fruits and vegetables studied, as well as being strongly cytotoxic against human leukemia cells. (Journal of Agriculture and Food Chemistry, 44:701-705; 3426-3343, 1996; 46:2686-2693, 1998).

Antioxidant activity is measured by ORAC, which stands for Oxygen Radical Absorbence Capacity. According to the U.S.D.A., these are the top ten:

1. Blueberries	47.0	6. Kiwis	6.0
2. Strawberries	15.4	7. Pink Grapefruit	4.8
3. Plums	9.5	8. White Grapes	4.5
4. Oranges	7.5	9. Bananas	2.2
5. Red Grapes	7.4	10. Apples	2.2

So the antioxidant activity of blueberries is 21 times that of apples, which nevertheless, contain other valuable nutrients, and are still good food!

Ronald L. Prior, Ph.D., at the Jean Mayer USDA Human Nutrition Center on Aging at Tufts University, concluded from this study that

---

"One-half cup of blueberries delivers as much antioxidant power as five servings of other fruits and vegetables — such as peas, carrots, apples, squash and broccoli."

James A. Joseph of the Human Nutrition Research Center on Aging reported in the <u>Journal of Neuroscience</u> that "age reversal" was actually occurring in a study in which rats were fed a powdered form of blueberries! After just eight weeks of giving rats blueberries, the 21 month old animals, which in terms of life span is on par with people in their late 60's, outperformed the *unsupplemented*, younger rats.

Joseph says, *"So, we got reversals in age-related declines."* The amount of blueberries that each animal ate, when adjusted for body weight, was equivalent to one cup daily in a person's diet, he notes.

U.S.D.A. research scientist, Dr. Richard Prior, states: *"As long as you're consuming oxygen, you need to be consuming antioxidants on a daily basis."* The best source is food, and secondarily, supplements that contain *whole* foods, not just isolated antioxidants that are synthetically derived in 99 percent of supplements.

I buy frozen blueberries and strawberries year round and eat some almost every day as one of the important deposits into my health account. I add them to my protein drink in the morning and to other foods such as cooked cereal.

For more information on "blueberry power", go to http://naturalhealthline.com/newsletter/990915/blueberries.htm on the web.

THE ESSENTIAL NUTRIENTS

The fifth critical element in the nutrition arena is making sure you are getting all the *essential* nutrients you need. What would your cake be like if you left out one of the critical ingredients? Using only 90 percent of the ingredients is not going to work well.

What nutrients are *essential*? We've known for decades that we need nutrients from three categories: protein, fat and carbohydrates.

Protein Power

What we really need from protein are the eight *essential* amino acids. Without all eight, we become ill and will not survive long because they are absolutely essential to our health. Eggs are one of the ideal sources of complete protein, notwithstanding the myth that they raise your cholesterol levels. This myth is based on studies done over 50 years ago—by the Cereal Industry! Those early studies used an *altered* food: dried egg yolk powder, not whole eggs. Dried egg yolk powder is a form of *oxidized* cholesterol, which as an *altered* food, as is most milk, is hard on your arteries. I have three eggs almost every morning, either raw in a protein drink or cooked. Cholesterol is not fat, and is an essential nutrient out of which your body makes hormones. 75 percent of your cholesterol is produced by your body. It only becomes a problem in the arteries when the body uses it to patch up the damage done in the arteries by free radicals, viruses and other toxic substances, such as chlorine.

Unaltered milk is good for some people, and a variety of fish and meat free of hormones and antibiotics is good as long as they are in balance with carbohydrates and fats, and not in excess. Beans, grains and seeds are also very important to include. It is best to have some protein with *every* meal (especially breakfast) based on the ideal ratio for your body type.

THE GOOD, BAD AND THE UGLY

We also need fat. Fat itself is good, and is not bad (unless it is altered by heating or hydrogenation). In fact, fat is *essential* and without it you'll become sick and die.

Eating food with fat is not inherently fattening.

Most of the extra fat people carry is from what their body made from excess sugar and refined carbohydrates.

The "ugly" fat is trans fat. This is ANY fat that has been *altered* by heating (stove top or deep fried), chemical processing or partial hydrogenation. These are deadly. The only good thing about these is that they are easy to identify and avoid if you stay on the lookout. Any *genetically* altered oil, such as rapeseed oil (renamed and known as Canola oil) would also fall into this category and should be avoided. "Ugly" fat that is most dangerous and the most ugly is any excess fat (from any source) you carry in or on your body.

"Bad" fat is getting *too much* of a good fat, such as saturated fats from dairy and meat, and from polyunsaturated omega 6 fats from vegetable oils (especially corn and canola). This is a mistake most people make.

The good fat is any fat other than trans fat that is in balance with the other kinds of fats. E.g. the monounsaturated fats from seeds, avocados, extra virgin olive oil and nuts are especially important.

Fat to the Rescue!

A recent study done at Emory University in Atlanta indicates that certain fats may ward off colon cancer. The June 1999 issue of the Journal of the American College of Nutrition reported that

LDL cholesterol fell 17 percent in people eating an almond-rich diet, but rose 2 percent in folks downing dairy-rich fare.

According to the British Medical Journal, a study done at the Harvard School of Public Health in Boston found that of the 86,000 women participating in the Nurses Health Study from 1980-1990, only 65 percent who ate at least 5 ounces of nuts a week were as likely to suffer heart disease, as compared to those who rarely ate nuts. Among nonsmoking teetotalers, it was only 50 percent.

There are three *essential* fatty acids. Many people lack one of the essential fatty acids called omega 3. The very *best* source of this is flaxseed or flaxseed oil. Salmon is another fairly good source.

A recent French study of 76,000 nurses concluded that consuming more omega 3 fat had reduced fatal heart attacks one third to one half.

Dr. Johanna Budwig, a seven time Nobel Prize nominee, is a world renown scientist and biochemist, and considered by many to be the foremost authority on fats and healing. One of her books is entitled, Flax Oil as a True Aid Against Arthritis, Heart Infraction, Cancer and other Diseases.

FIGHTING FAT WITH FAT

Sometimes you need to fight fire with fire. One way to fight fat is with fat. Eliminating all fat from your diet is a misguided strategy that will backfire on you by creating the opposite results of what you want. Refined carbohydrates and high glycemic index foods are easily converted to fat, and if you are lacking certain essential fat in your diet, even a higher percentage will be converted to and stored as fat.

The identity of the "fat hero" is flaxseed or flaxseed oil as your best source of Omega-3 fatty acids. Flaxseed oil has been called an "anti-fat" fat because it helps your body burn fat more efficiently. Flaxseed oil is converted to compounds that stoke the metabolic processes of the cells. Much like a furnace that is stoked, cells generate more heat and burn fuel faster with flaxseed oil. Ann Louise Gittleman, author of Your Body Knows Best, goes so far as to say that *"any weight loss program undertaken without the addition of the essential nutrients in flaxseed oil is destined to fail."*

For a free sample of Flaxseed oil, go to www.barleans.com or call (800) 445-3529.

Personally, I eat some raw nuts (almonds and cashews) and seeds (sunflower, pumpkin and flax) every day, plus Flaxseed oil. I consider these to be an essential daily deposit into my health account. I recommend that you do too.

SUPER SUGARS

Carbohydrate technology is the arena in which there have been the most recent and exciting breakthroughs. In fact, this next section may be the most important part of this book for you, because, like many people, you may see the most rapid and dramatic differences when you begin including the *missing* "super carbohydrates" or "super sugars" into your diet.

All people who incorporate the essential "super sugars" into their diets begin receiving significant health benefits within 24 hours. Sometimes people experience dramatic results the very first day, whereas for others, improvement may not be obvious for several days, weeks and sometimes even months.

Until about ten years ago, research scientists and thus doctors, believed that the *only* function of sugar and carbohydrates (which breaks down into simple sugars), was to provide energy. The fact that there were over two hundred simple sugars (saccharides) in nature appeared irrelevant.

But now it has been confirmed that carbohydrates do far more than provide energy—they are essential components of the cell to cell communication, which in turn is ESSENTIAL for the immune system function and all other systems in your body.

The 24th edition of a medical text called Harper's Biochemistry (Murray et al., 1996) first alerted the medical schools and public to at least eight known and specific saccharides (sugars) that are involved in the communication and intracellular function of virtually all the cells in the body.

Scientists now know that there are *eight essential sugars*. <u>Harper's Biochemistry</u> lists these as galactose, glucose, mannose, fucose (*not* fructose), *N*-acetylneuraminic acid, *N*-acetygalactosamine acid, *N*-acetyglucosamine and Xylose.

These simple sugars (saccharides) are absolutely necessary for <u>cell to cell communication</u>, which help the body stay healthy.

Internal Civil War

Here's how the Spring/Summer 1999 issue of <u>Newsweek</u> magazine described the disruption of cell to cell communication in auto-immune diseases:

"Healthy immune systems work around the clock to fight off viruses and bacteria. T cells, the soldiers of the body, monitor for foreign invaders or antigens. When necessary, they call out the troops—an army of B cells—to destroy the enemy. But in people with auto-immune diseases, the T cells go hay-wire: <u>they somehow become confused, mistaking the self for an outsider and assaulting healthy tissue</u>."

Within the next several years, the critical role of the essential sugars, which are also known as glyconutrients, will become common knowledge among both doctors and the general public. It is already beginning to happen! It is expected that someday glyconutrients will become "standard of care" by medical doctors for all auto-immune diseases, just like penicillin is standard of care for infections and chemotherapy for cancer. In fact, doctors can be held liable for malpractice if they do not use "standard of care" treatment for the appropriate disease.

The Missing Pieces to the Puzzle?

The bad news is that we are only getting two of the essential eight sugars in our food. This is evidently one of the major contributing factors to our declining immune system function and the corresponding dramatic increase in disease. To illustrate, if your eight-cylinder car had only two cylinders running, how far would it go and how well would it work? It is imperative that you get the other missing six sugars (saccharides).

HEALTH INSURANCE YOU CAN EAT

The good news is that there is a way to get all eight essential sugars, either individually or as a complete glyconutrient complex. For thousands of people, getting all eight essential sugars in a glyconutrient complex has felt like experiencing a miracle. And unlike common sugar (high glycemic index) which stresses the pancreas and can be particularly damaging for diabetics, glyconutrients (low glycemic index) do not have this adverse effect.

Fortunately, because these essential sugars are *so important*, our bodies were designed to be able to synthesize the missing six, as long as we weren't overloaded with toxins and stress, and had all the other proper nutrients. But, with severely depleted soil, over-processed food, a heavily polluted and toxic environment, and stress added on top, our bodies just cannot do it efficiently.

Medical Breakthrough of the Century?

A growing number of scientists and doctors around the world, such as Dr. Steve Nugent, consider the development of a glyconutrient complex that contains all eight essential sugars as the "medical breakthrough of the century."

In fact, the 1999 Nobel Prize in Medicine was awarded to Dr. Guenter Blobel for discovering how glyconutrients function as address tags for directing the delivery of proteins to the proper location in cells. This is cellular communication.

Modulate vs. Stimulate

As an immune system *modulator*, glyconutrients do not *stimulate* the immune system or *do anything to* your body, unlike drugs which force a biochemical reaction. Instead, glyconutrients give your body what's been *missing* so that your body can do whatever is most appropriate—either boost the immune system function (up to 400 percent) or modulate it down if it is overactive as it is in allergies, asthma, lupus and most auto-immune diseases.

According to Dr. Darryl See, M.D., *"There has been no other substance in the history of medicine that has achieved immune system modulation."*

Because many conditions such as asthma, diabetes, heart disease, lupus, etc. have BOTH under-active and overactive elements of immune system function, the availability of an immune system modulator is a very significant breakthrough.

Here's the perspective of Michael D. Schlachter, MD, Board Certified Internal Medicine and Pulmonary Disease:

"The use of glyconutrients in my practice of medicine has become so second nature, that to care for patients without it would be like trying to perform surgery without a scalpel. It has become an integral part of utilizing the body's ability to heal itself along with heightening the effects of pharmaceuticals when needed."

When "miracles" happen, remember that the healing is not from a powder or capsule but from the body being able to heal itself when it has all it needs, as it was designed to do.

DR. SEE'S LANDMARK STUDY

The most significant and comprehensive *In Vitro* screening study to date was published in the <u>Journal of the American Nutraceutical Association</u> on "196 Natural Products for Toxicity and Efficacy." This was a six-year study funded partially by a grant from the National Institutes of Health for a study on

Fibromyalgia. It was done at the University of California in Irvine, by Dr. Darryl See, one of the top immunologists in the world. Some of the results have also been published in the American Journal of Natural Medicine, vol. 5 #6, 1998, p10; Integrative Physiological and Behavioral Science, vol. 33 #3, 1998, p 280; and Immunopharmacology vol. 35, 1997, p.229. Additionally, portions of these astounding research results were presented at a UCI Medical School Department of Medicine-sponsored "Grand Rounds".

What he discovered was quite surprising. Of the 196 natural products tested (450 nutrients from 57 different companies), 49.9 percent showed liver or blood toxicity and potential drug interactions. These were all natural products that are touted to be the best products available, including all the other popular saccharide products like those from the noni plant, aloe vera, echinacea and glucosamine which gave only moderate stimulation to natural killer cell production of about 10 to 15%.

All 196 products were also tested in three areas of efficacy: antiviral effects, enhancement of natural killer cells and antioxidant activity as measured by raising glutathione levels.

Only five of the 196 were significantly effective in all three efficacy parameters with no toxicity in the other three parameters tested.

Wonder what the top five were? Fourth and fifth place were garlic and fresh (not processed) aloe vera. The top three were glyconutrient complexes, based on the new cutting-edge carbohydrate technology.

Another remarkable distinction of glyconutrients is that they also have the additional benefit of creating a dramatic antioxidant effect in the body far beyond any of the more commonly used antioxidants.

The primary defense against oxidative stress or rusting inside the cell is a substance called glutathione. Glyconutrients vastly increase glutathione levels, therefore decreasing oxidative stress and the rusting of the inside of the cell.

An Historical First

According to Dr. Darryl See, "...*glyconutritionals are the ONLY substance in the history of medicine that has ever been discovered that takes care of both of the mechanisms of chronic diseases in a totally non-toxic manner. First, oxidative stress or rusting of the cells, and also immune system dysfunction.*"

Doctor Robert Ortmann is an immunologist and a research scientist from the National Institutes of Health in Bethesda, Maryland, which is probably the leading, most respected research center in the world.

Here is Dr. Ortmann's perspective on glyconutrients: (this does not constitute an endorsement by the National Institutes of Health):

> "*I really believe that they are something that is going to be mandatory for overall general health, and the reason I have come to these conclusions is because I have spent the past several months doing what I call research on the research. And when I would do searches on glyconutrients, and especially a lot of different disease processes, I was just floored by the number of quality studies that are out there that have shown such benefit and promise in a myriad of diseases ranging from diabetes to arthritis.*
>
> "*I believe that glyconutrients are going to become a staple nutritional supplement for all six billion people on the face of this earth within the next two to five years.*"

Because I continue to see incredible results for both myself and others, I will be taking glyconutrients for the rest of my life. If you are committed to having vibrant health and longevity, I strongly recommend that you do so as well.

This is "health insurance you can eat" and one of the most important deposits you can make on a daily basis into your health account.

Understand though, no supplements will ever *cure* any disease—they simply play an essential *role* in supporting the immune system which does the healing.

Richard Cannon, a professional biologist in Alaska, wanted to know why these glyconutrients had made such a significant improvement in his health. So he searched the published scientific literature and compiled much of it on www.hometown.aol.com/r4cannon. You will find it very educational.

What is Your Real Age?

There are three valid ways to measure your age. Your chronological age is how old you are by the calendar. Your biological age is the age of your body in terms of critical life signs, organ function and cellular processes. Your psychological age is based on how old you feel. All three are important and valid, but only the first one is fixed. The other two can be reversed.

There are eighty year olds who are younger *biologically* than some twenty-five year olds. In fact, diabetes is considered to be a condition of accelerated aging.

Scientists have discovered a way to measure your health, or biological age, by using ten biomarkers. According to the book, Biomarkers—The 10 Strategies to Prolonging Vitality, by William Evans, Ph.D. and Irwin Rosenberg, M.D., the ten biomarkers are:

Lean body (muscle) mass
Strength
Basal metabolic rate
Body fat percentage
Insulin sensitivity
Aerobic capacity
Blood pressure

Cholesterol/HDL ratio
Bone density
Body temperature regulation

Note that at least half of these (the first five) biomarkers are enhanced by eating foods with a low glycemic index.

The first nine of these biomarkers now have studies to support that the use of glyconutrients can actually *reverse* that biomarker, and the tenth one has strong preliminary evidence to support reversal on it, also.

TRAINS NEED FUEL!

This fifth strategy, based on the Wood dynamic, is about nourishment. This is the final piece in our train analogy.

Your train needs fuel! It needs the *proper* fuel for your train. If your train is designed to run on wood or coal, using oil will not work very well.

Your body, being a million times more sophisticated than a train, needs certain high quality nourishment, certain ratios, a lot of variety and specific essential nutrients. Any old fuel will not do for your body, even though it may seem to run even on junk fuel (this is because the body can compensate, sometimes for a long time, before it inevitably breaks down).

So just being on the right track (purpose—Fire dynamic), being well-connected (Earth dynamic) to the tracks, other cars and your crew, avoiding the dangers of rocks (Metal dynamic), and moving (Water dynamic) is not enough. You need to keep supplying your train with the proper fuel! Otherwise, your mission will fail.

But with the proper dynamics (Fire, Earth, Metal, Water and Wood) your train can go for many more decades and your body can prevent and/or cure any disease and enjoy vibrant health, happiness and longevity!

For a FREE health analysis on this or the other four health strategies, go to www.cureanydisease.com and download the

WELLdisk for free, or request the WELLdisk ($10 value) as a free gift by calling (888) 666-8942 or (800) 700-1238 (small shipping charge applies).

Miracle Stories

Kathy Smith ~ Hepatitis, Cancer, Colitis, Crohn's Disease

My health problems started at age fifteen when I contracted a strange kind of hepatitis. There was no name for it and it was not contagious. I had it a total of three times. The doctors told my parents I would not live through my teen years.

I have continued to be plagued with health problems even though I used all kinds of supplements and ate a good diet. I even grew most of my own vegetables and used mostly organic meats. I searched for years for something to help my body gain health and spent lots and lots of money on it.

In the late '80s and early '90s I developed ulcerative colitis along with Crohn's disease and developed a sudden hearing loss. Then in 1997, I was diagnosed with one of the most aggressive cancers there is. I did not go to an oncologist because I knew what he would want to do. Sadly, I watched both of my parents die of cancer. I knew the regular conventional way was not the way to go. I had it in the intestines, liver, kidneys, and adrenals.

In November of 1997, I was introduced to the strategies for vibrant health. From November 1997 to April 1998, I no longer had any cancer. Even with the strategies it was not easy. In April 1999, I again was diagnosed with cancer starting in the intestines. At this time I had been in contact with Dr. John Branden who uses the strategies. He suggested changes in my program. By July 1999, I was once again cancer free.

Stephanie Reed ~ Asthma, Allergies, Endometriosis; Weight Loss, Cancer

I believe the most significant starting point for this story is when I was eighteen and began taking tetracycline to treat acne. By my mid-twenties I had developed allergies (to most pollens), asthma, and endometriosis. I had begun taking antihistamines and decongestants by my mid-twen-

ties and when the endometriosis became apparent, I took Tylenol 3 for a few days each month. This period of time was the beginning of my reliance on prescription drugs and, consequently, the rapid accumulation of toxins. The tetracycline was certainly quite effective at reducing my good bacteria levels, allowing candida yeast to rage out of control. I believe this probably played a major role in my health for many years to come.

At age thirty-one I had a complete hysterectomy, which then meant taking estrogen. At age thirty-eight (1987) I was diagnosed with breast cancer and had to immediately discontinue taking estrogen permanently. This meant a sudden, premature menopause. I took large amounts of progestin (Provera) to control the unbearable night sweats, but it caused numerous side effects. But the alternative was virtually not sleeping, so I used the only tool I knew of to simply get by in life.

After the mastectomy in 1987, I suffered from esophagitis, apparently as a result of excess radiation therapy. To try to cope with the continuous heartburn, I began taking an acid reducer (Zantac). I was unable to eat most fruits and vegetables as well as anything acid or spicy. With this very limited diet I developed an extreme dairy allergy.

In 1990 I was found to have had significant bone mass loss and began treatment, which meant taking the drug Didronel and additional calcium supplements.

My allergies overall were worsening. I gained sixty-five pounds and my blood pressure was running in the range of 140-170/ to 90-106. I was finally realizing that the doctors had nothing further to offer me and gave me no hope that I would get off any of the drugs. This was apparently as good as it was going to get — and that was a dismal realization.

In 1993 I was introduced to herbs. Being skeptical, I had to be educated and given convincing, reliable evidence of safety and effectiveness before plunging in to this different approach. The herbs were helpful, but after awhile I found that I had reached the limit of their benefits. At this point I was introduced to the strategies for vibrant health by a friend.

Within a few weeks I no longer was having hot flashes, halved the tetracycline and antihistamine/decongestant, and discontinued the Zantac and Didronel. (After six years of treatment for the bone density loss, I was lower than where I had started; so the conclusion was that the treatment was ineffective.) I noticed I was losing significant inches, *although I hadn't actually lost weight. I was feeling great!*

After about four months I decided to more aggressively deal with the huge candida yeast overgrowth. A few weeks later my allergies were noticeably reduced and I was also able to completely discontinue the tetracycline. After a total of about ten months, I was completely off the antihistamine/decongestant which was the last of the prescription drugs. That was July of 1997, and up until now (July 1999) I have not taken any kind of drugs. That is quite an accomplishment!

My 1997 bone density scans indicated my spine was 78 percent of normal for my age and my hip was 88 percent of normal. In May 1999, a heel scan indicated I am now at 108 percent of normal. During 1997 I had body scans five months apart and during that time there was a decrease in body fat of 3 percent and an even bigger gain in lean tissue. I can see and feel much more improvement since then, reflecting a much improved body composition.

In May 1998, I began having colon hydrotherapy to help speed up the removal of the candida. While I had not thought I had any bowel problems, it is clear that I needed some help in removing some of the toxic buildup. This also uncovered two different parasites that I did not know I had. Going through the colonics has encouraged me to modify my diet more significantly, and the cleansing process has allowed my nutrients to be absorbed better; so my progress has become quite obvious as I have now lost forty-five pounds since beginning the strategies.

Since using these strategies that a friend introduced to me, I have continually been losing inches, whether or not my weight was decreasing. Interestingly, when I was last at my current weight, just prior to the mastectomy, I was two dress sizes larger. This has been an almost unbelievable process.

I should also mention that my blood tests have been reflecting continual improvements. I am looking so good in so many ways that I still sometimes have a hard time comprehending what I have accomplished. My blood pressure is now 110/70. My DHEA (hormones) level has gone from less than 16 percent to 67 percent, which was my ultimate goal. Most of that change occurred during 1998. I have no signs of any allergies - - and they had ruled my life for over twenty years. I don't remember when I had so much energy. I look healthier in so many ways that everyone wants to know what I have been doing.

They keep repeating how GREAT I am looking.

I never expected to be off the drugs and had given up on losing the weight and thought I would never enjoy many foods that most people take for granted. Since I have worked hard to get to where I am today, I am not interested in reverting back to old habits; so indulging in some of these foods is an occasional treat. But that in itself is a giant reward. I know that with the strategies coupled with the desire to take responsibility for our health that virtually anyone can greatly enhance their quality of life. I'm feeling younger all the time - and you can too!

Barbara Tompkins ~ Panic Attacks, Arthritis pain

I am semi-retired but work for the Clark County School District as a substitute teacher for disabled children. Before I was introduced to the strategies for vibrant health, I suffered with panic attacks to such a degree that I was afraid to go out by myself. For two and a half years I did not drive. I saw doctors and a psychiatrist for my condition. The psychiatrist wanted to put me on drugs so that I could live a normal life without the fear of going out alone. I refused to take the drugs.

My beauty operator, Doris Diaz, introduced me to the strategies in October of 1997. I started using them around the seventh of October and in a couple of months I was feeling good, had more energy, and as time went by, I noticed other things, like not having any arthritic pain in my shoulders and wrists. The most important thing is that I have not had a panic attack since November of 1997. I could finally feel free to go out by myself and I went back to work in January of this year. I am no longer afraid.

Kerri Hutton-Hermez ~ Hypoglycemia, Irritable bowel, Fibromyalgia, PMS, Bladder Infections

I am a single mother of four, and about twenty years ago I began a long, hopeless slide downhill. Over that twenty years, I had been diagnosed with multiple conditions and diseases- - none of which could be cured and all that worsened as time went on.

I was plagued with hypoglycemia, irritable bowel (that was accompanied by fainting one to two times daily because of pain),

Haashimoto disease, Raynaud's, severe and worsening premenstrual syndrome, migraines, irritable bladder and multiple bladder infections, indigestion, excessive gas and bloating, and after years of being fatigued all day, not sleeping well at night, zero energy, depression, dizziness, excessive and ongoing pain in fourteen sites on my body, I was finally diagnosed with fibromyalgia.

Refusing the traditional course of treatment - - painkillers, anti-inflammatories, and antidepressants - - which have gruesome long-term side effects, I spent my days in pain. I felt frustrated and hopeless about my future and that of my children. At the time, my youngest was only six months!

Just when I thought it could not get much worse, a doctor advised me that according to the latest test results, I seemed to be headed for lupus or even possibly multiple sclerosis.

My cousins shared the strategies of vibrant health with me. At that point I would have tried anything. At the end of two weeks I felt something—nothing specific - - but something which was more positive than I had felt for years.

At the end of six weeks I could go up and down the stairs to my bathroom without being absolutely breathless and in severe pain. I just got better from there. Today I run and play with my kids, work two jobs, and make plans for our future. I love to tell my story to anyone who will listen, particularly those without help and hope like I once was.

Doris Chabot ~ Back Pain, Chronic Hip Pain, Polio, PMS, Pain, Fatigue

I had polio when I was four years old, have always had back pain, and spent numerous hours throughout my life in doctors' offices, physiotherapy, message therapy, etc. I had scoliosis and chronic hip pain. About fifteen years ago I also had serious premenstrual syndrome symptoms, hypothyroidism, and increasing overall pain in my body.

I hated going to doctors and always felt like a chronic complainer. Usually I would be given pain pills, anti-inflammatory pills, Valium, and antidepressants. I developed serious ulcers and couldn't eat a lot of things.

I had been a secretary, but the pain of sitting all day drove me crazy. I decided to go to college and when trying to figure out what career path to pursue, the primary factor in my decision was to find a career where I would be moving around a lot. The basis of my career choice was how to deal with the pain.

I have had several gastroscopies, sigmoidoscopies, biopsies, and various other stomach tests as the doctors thought I might have stomach cancer. I was also given antibiotics and ulcer medication such as Tagamet. I took those for a long time.

About ten years ago I was diagnosed with candida and fibromyalgia. The doctors didn't know what to do and so I went to a naturopath. I worked diligently on dietary changes and was able to cure the candida and most of the PMS symptoms, but I still had pain everywhere. By this time, due to all the stomach problems and the fear of stomach cancer, I refused to take any pharmaceuticals and decided that I should just learn to live with this, and I did. I was resigned to a life of pain and adjusted accordingly.

I continued to work. I had to give up almost everything else as I had no energy. I rarely went out. I didn't go to movies because I couldn't sit there that long. I didn't go to church or concerts, for the same reasons. Even though I only had enough income to maintain myself, I learned that there were things I couldn't do so I had to pay people to accomplish some of the more physical tasks such as shoveling and lawn mowing.

I could only vacuum one room at a time, and then rest. My washer and dryer are in the basement and I only went down once a week to do laundry and often stayed down there the whole time as stairs were becoming more difficult to do. But most of all I had little energy to do anything. I had previously been a very neat person, and found my house to be more and more messy. I just couldn't keep up so I learned to live with the mess.

One of the most frustrating things with fibromyalgia and chronic fatigue syndrome is that I was having more and more trouble concentrating and remembering anything. I was so scared because I thought I was getting early Alzheimer's. I was also scared because I wondered how I would live if I couldn't work as I am alone. I knew I had to work but I was spending more and more money getting people to do things around my house. I got very depressed, suicidal, and felt very hopeless. No one seemed to know what to do.

I quit going to the doctor and just dealt with my general practition-

er who was kind and helpful but who didn't really know what to do about the pain. She sent me to a vericose vein doctor even though I didn't have any visible vericose veins, because the pain in my legs and feet was becoming unbearable. I was told I didn't have any internal type of vericose veins and that the pain was probably just the fibromyalgia. I am very grateful to this doctor as she put up with my negative moods, and tried everything she could.

Then life got worse. I lost several aunts and uncles to cancer in a year, then my mom was diagnosed with cancer, and then I lost my job. As soon as I heard about my mom, a friend told me about the strategies for vibrant health. Mom died three weeks later so it was probably too late anyway. So I decided to try the strategies myself. Within four days the brain fog lifted and I could think straight for the first time in a long time. The correcting crisis lasted about three weeks. I noticed that the pain in my neck had lessened. Then a few weeks later, the pain in my shoulders lessened, and eventually my feet and legs also felt better. Prior to this, I was wearing support socks all the time and I had my feet up on a desk whenever I could. Needless to say, this was a great improvement.

Now I go up and down stairs about ten times a day, I can mow the whole lawn at once and clean the flower beds and do a whole day of yard work without feeling exhausted.

The greatest benefit, of course, is that the pain is gone. I am calm and can take things in stride. My outlook is much more positive whereas before all I envisioned for my future was to save money so I could move to a one level house and pay for people to look after me. I thought about suicide a lot. My entire life is better.

Eric ~ Asthma, Cleft Lip, Allergies, Lupus

My son Eric had his first asthma attack at 12 weeks old. He was born a very toxic little boy, having a cleft lip and many food allergies and allergies to medications. It seemed like every three weeks or so I would bring him to the emergency room to get him stronger medication as the stuff we had at home was not working. After two years of this I was pretty exhausted. My sister Laurie, who has Lupus, got such great results using the principles of vibrant health we decided to try them on Eric.

Wow! The first thing we noticed was his pale, milky skin and large purple circles under his eyes disappeared. He was very little and in the first year he grew about 7 inches. The scar from his cleft lip is barely visible now. In the last 2 years he has used his asthma medication 3 times. Thanks to these strategies, my son can enjoy a normal, happy, and healthy life.

Elaine Tipton ~ Colon Cancer

Four years ago I had a tumor the size of my fist removed along with about two feet of my colon. I went to Mexico for treatment hoping to avoid the standard year of chemotherapy they were recommending here. The doctor there said because of the type of cancer, he would also recommend chemo along with their alternative treatment of over seventy capsules of supplements/vitamins per day. I took the chemo for about six months, finishing up in April of 1996. I stayed on their supplements and vitamins but gradually was getting toxic to some of them. I was getting depressed, my liver just could not filter it all, and my skin was an absolute mess. My skin was so dry I remember waking up each morning clawing at my legs, they itched so bad.

In February of 1997 I started the strategies for vibrant health based on a friend's advice. Within a week, my legs started healing. My far-sightedness has improved. I am doing so much better and feel healthy for the first time in years.

Lou Ledger ~ Lupus, High Blood Pressure

About fourteen years ago, I began experiencing pain around the joints in my hands, arms, shoulders, knees, hips, and ankles. Gradually over a period of several months, I began to lose much of the use of my hands and arms. This caused me a lot of pain to the point that I had to have help doing the most basic things, such as dressing myself, combing my hair, and many other personal things. Thank the Lord for an understanding and most helpful husband who cared for me.

I finally went to the doctor who diagnosed what I had as lupus and put me on Prednisone. It helped but I was afraid of what it was doing to my body.

I started the strategies for vibrant health about four months later which I heard about from a friend and I began to wean myself from the Prednisone. When I no longer had to take that, I began to notice that my blood pressure was lower and that my heartbeat was more regular. I talked with my doctor and told her what I was doing and how I was feeling. At this point, I have had no prescription medication for approximately four and a half months and I'm doing great!

Ron Yates ~ Mood Swings, Allergies, Alcoholism

Within a week of trying the strategies to health I was off Prozac, a drug I had been taking for about two years because of mood swings. Additionally, I noticed my allergies completely disappeared. I have also experienced problems with alcoholism and after four months using the strategies, my craving for alcohol has diminished considerably. For the first time in over thirty years I can choose water over alcohol without much effort. Along with a new, almost unexplainable feeling of well-being, I truly feel in control of my life again!

8

PLAYING THE
WHOLE TEAM

Maximizing Your Results

Life in Five Chapters

Miracle Stories

Maximizing Your Results

To get the full long-term value of any of these five strategies, you need to incorporate *all five* of them into your life. You may see good results with one or two, but you will see *phenomenal* results when you have the synergistic effect of all five working in concert, just as the five players on a basketball team have success only when playing together. So if you want a winning season, make sure you are using all five players!

There are three very powerful ways to accelerate your velocity on your freeway to vibrant health and longevity.

Your First Step

One is to make a solid commitment to doing all you can to achieve your health freedom. Put this in writing.

It's imperative that you get very clear to what you are most committed: immediate pleasure and convenience (which only has *short* term benefits), OR to your life and health freedom with *long* term benefits such as vibrant health, happiness and longevity.

Also record your answers to these four powerful questions:

> **1. WHY?** Why do you want to enjoy vibrant health, happiness and longevity? In what ways would your life be different? To which people would it matter the most, e.g. your spouse, children or grandchildren? Be very specific and detailed. This should be at least one page, but the longer the better.

> **2. WHY NOT?** Why not go for health freedom and vibrant health? Why not beat the odds? Are there any good reasons not to make the commitment, e.g. could you lose your disability income? Would people give you less attention? Are you afraid to face the possibility of failing? Would someone, even perhaps a doctor, belittle or mock

you for doing something "ridiculous" by taking the "road less traveled"?

3. WHY NOT YOU? Others have achieved what some considered to be impossible—why not you? Others have broken through the deadly barrier of doubt and hopelessness—why not you? Others have had "miracles"—why not you? Others have achieved and now enjoy vibrant health, happiness and longevity—why not you?

4. WHY NOT NOW? Is there a better time to start than now? Is there really something more important than taking time to go after your health freedom? Why not now?

Now make a decision to read your answers to these four important questions every day and add to your journal how you are doing and feeling daily. Express your fears, anger, doubts, and of course, your faith, as weak as it may be that day. Record and celebrate every time you notice an improvement. Expect and track your progress.

Then go public with your decision. Share your answers to the above four questions with someone you trust. This can strengthen your resolve and faith. If some well-meaning people try to convince you that you are not being realistic, thank them for their concern and opinion but don't listen to them. Find at least one person who can stand with you in your faith for vibrant health and longevity, who will encourage and build you up if you get discouraged.

Your Second Step

The second way to accelerate your velocity on your freeway to vibrant health and longevity is to practice *each* of the five strategies (Fire, Earth, Metal, Water and Wood) every day. It is imperative that you do this with the *specific intention and purpose of achieving your specific written health goals* as opposed to doing the right things just because they are good for you in general.

For example, if one of your goals is to have normal and stable blood sugar (you're currently diabetic), then when you drink water, eat good food, do your movements or exercise, or take essential nutrients, do it with the *specific purpose and intention* of achieving your goal of normal stable blood sugar.

Keep a daily record of how well you are doing in each of the five strategies. Do this by recording a number (using a scale from one to ten, ten being the highest) that best describes how you did in each of the five strategies for that day. (Your score would be 50 points if you gave yourself a ten in each category.) Then double that number to convert it to a percentage, and see how close you get to 100 each day.

Your Third Step—The Appreciation Dynamic

The third powerful way to accelerate progress toward health freedom is *appreciation*. YOU MUST NOT UNDERESTIMATE THE POWER OF FEELING APPRECIATION FROM YOUR HEART!

Use this in many ways. Feel from your heart a deep sense of appreciation every time you do something to support and enhance your health, especially as you eat your supplements.

Take a block of time (five to ten minutes) each day to feel appreciation and gratitude from your heart for one or more people (this could include God). This is especially important to do at the beginning of the day and at the end of each day.

Throughout each day you also can practice feeling appreciation for each person with whom you interact.

The more you experience appreciation *from your heart*, the more you will dramatically strengthen your immune system.

This effect can be easily measured with modern heart monitoring equipment. In fact, focusing on your heart and feeling appreciation for a block of fifteen minutes will have an electronically measurable significant benefit for four hours!

Appreciate yourself and your body; appreciate whatever you are doing at the moment to attain vibrant health. Be grateful to God who designed your body with the capacity to recover and be healthy.

Like salt that enhances the taste of food, adding a heart-felt appreciation to any deposit you make into your health account can double or triple the credit to your account and move you faster towards achieving your goals.

Also, have an appreciation for any health problem that you currently have instead of resenting it. Do this by seeing it as your body's best attempt to compensate for and manage all the stress and issues it has to handle, including toxins and insufficient nourishment.

For more invaluable information on this powerful technology developed by scientific researchers, acquire the Heart Math material at heartmath.com or by calling (800) 700-1238 or (888) 666-8942.

"I'm Fading Fast!"

If you have a serious, life-threatening problem, you need to do three additional things.

First, be sure you are well connected with people who care about you, especially with at least one person who believes with you that you can restore and recover your health.

Second, it is important that you access the perspective of a professional, holistically minded healthcare provider whom you can trust, whether an MD, naturopath, nutritionist, chiropractor, kinesiologist, Acupuncturist, etc.

Third, it is advisable to do EVERYTHING you can, not just a few things. Reread this book, read other books and do *everything* you can to recover your health. You will need more than the maintenance dosage of supplements, in some cases ten to twenty times as much.

"Who Ya Gonna Call?"

If you need specific professional advice on what supplements can help you most for your condition and how much to take, contact the Pharmacist Health Network at www.callpne.com to schedule an appointment or call 888-388-5522 or 900-CALLP-NE. Also, if a friend gave you or told you about this book, they may know of other resources as well.

Most of the books and resources mentioned are available from (800) 700-1238 or (888) 666-8942.

LIFE IN FIVE CHAPTERS

If you are really ready to commit to changing your life and habits so that you can enjoy vibrant health and longevity, there are usually five stages through which you need to go, as described by Sufi poet Rumi:

Chapter One: I walk down the street. There's a deep hole in the sidewalk. I fall in. I am lost; I am hopeless; it isn't my fault, and it takes forever to find a way out.

Chapter Two: I walk down the same street. There's a deep hole in the sidewalk; I pretend I don't see it; I fall in. I can't believe I'm in the same place again! It isn't my fault, and it still takes a long time to get out.

Chapter Three: I walk down the street, the same street. There's a deep hole in the sidewalk. I see it is there, and I still fall in. It's a habit; my eyes are open; I know where I am. It is my fault, and I get out immediately.

Chapter Four: I walk down the same street. There's a deep hole in the sidewalk. I walk around it.

Chapter Five: I walk down a different street and warn others to avoid the street with the deep hole in the sidewalk.

Be patient with yourself. Rome was not built in a day; nor can you change everything at once. Changing, even for the better, even when your life and health is at stake, can be difficult and takes time to fully accomplish. Appreciate where you are right now, appreciate your efforts and struggles, as well as the direction in which you are now headed. Be patient with yourself and others. Allow some time for change to occur, but just don't take too long—too much is at stake!

Miracle Stories

Greg Morrisson ~ Son's Autism
My husband and I had our world turned upside down after our son was diagnosed with autism. Our two-and-a-half-year-old son, Marshall, was a typical little boy who started changing and became developmentally delayed after his one year and eighteen month immunizations.

Marshall went from a happy, affectionate little boy to a very distant child who would have nothing to do with his family. He would bang his head when angry and cry in the corner with his blankie. He wouldn't allow us to hold or cuddle him. He developed lots of tactile sensitivities, became a very picky eater, and stopped trying to talk.

We noticed changes when we tried the strategies for vibrant health December 1996 after a friend introduced us to them. The change I noticed the most started on Christmas Day when Marshall lay down beside me and let me cuddle him for about half an hour. That was the best Christmas present I got. As time went by he became more and more cuddly and is now an affectionate little boy again.

Marshall is still non-verbal but chatters and sings all the time and is constantly learning new sounds and trying to say some words. He still has lots of sensitivities. At the rate he is learning, we feel he will soon be talking. He is still behind but catching up fast and we have high hopes for him going to a regular class in school in the future.

Jill Shirk ~ Damage from Radiation Treatment
We want to share an incredible story of Jill's transformed health, which began about two and one half years ago. At the time, she had endured sixteen years of failing health which followed treatment for cancer. We are thankful her treatment stopped her cancer, but in the process it severely damaged her health.

Some of the problems she experienced are heart-wrenching. Radiation destroyed her thyroid which resulted in the need for a synthetic medication. Sometimes the dosage was too much (with hyper days and sleepless nights), and sometimes too little (with no energy). Radiation also apparently scarred her spinal cord, for she was only able to walk for about fifteen to twenty minutes before her legs would go numb. She endured flu-like pain in all her joints and muscles that gradually worsened. Headaches became so painful that she often took as many as two or three prescribed capsules each day for the last four or five years.

Jill tried the strategies for vibrant health that a friend told us about. One Sunday morning, two weeks later, Jill was suddenly aware of a very strange feeling. She said, "For the first time since my cancer, I was aware that I felt quiet inside. I don't know how to describe it, but all those years I felt like there was a war going on inside of me and now it's all quiet and I don't hurt anywhere!"

Almost every day after that she began to notice new health improvements, and after two months she said, "Today, all those problems I suffered for sixteen years are almost entirely gone! I don't hurt anywhere, my full strength and stamina have returned, my headaches are gone, I no longer need the nasal inhaler, and my nose has healed. The day after Christmas (sixty days after starting the strategies) my husband and I walked for eight hours at South Coast Plaza (a shopping mall), and my legs did not go numb. However, neither of us noticed until we returned to the car. When we finally realized this, tears welled in both of our eyes.

Kate Jackson ~ Perimenopause, Migraines, Weight

Each month I suffered more and more prior to each menstrual cycle. I had night sweats, hot flashes, mood swings, itchy skin, insomnia, and horrendous headaches. Before the onset of each period I would get a migraine that sent me to bed for several days. Since my cycle was about every three weeks, I was miserable, in pain, and unable to take care of my family for three days every three weeks. This was not a happy time.

In January 1996 things hit an all-time low. One migraine was so intense it caused me to vomit. My husband took me to the doctor, who gave me a shot of Demerol and prescribed pain medication. That was *all! My husband and I went back to the doctor and begged him for hormone replacement therapy (HRT). The HRT (estrogen and proges-terone) relieved the migraines; however, over the next few months I began gaining weight, felt lethargic, and was unhappy with myself. I knew my body was not in balance.*

In May friends of ours told us about the strategies to health. Although my husband felt better immediately, it took me about a month to notice some improvement (realize I was still taking hormones). After three months my food cravings had diminished and I decided to wean myself off the synthetic hormones (HRT). I did, and have not experienced any of my menopausal symptoms, including the headaches. And my periods began to stretch out to longer intervals.

What a joy it is to have the strategies for vibrant health. I have gradually lost some of that extra weight and feel more energetic.

David and JoAnn Young ~ Candida around the heart; Weight loss, Low Energy

After we were told that my husband, David had candida around the heart, we started the strategies for vibrant health that a friend told us about. The doctor said my husband could potentially die of a heart attack. Needless to say, after being married only one year and having a brand new baby, this news was devastating. He was put on a candi-da cleanse and we did not see a lot of difference until he used the strategies along with it. The cleanse immediately kicked in and he had amazing improvements! His energy level is through the roof and his resistance to viruses is way up.

In the process of getting my husband's health on track, I started to notice that my energy went way up! I was also beginning to lose the weight that I had been trying so hard to lose after our baby was born.

Cindy Schattenkirk ~ Fibromyalgia

I had gone to the doctor for many years and could feel myself getting more and more run down. My doctor really did not know what to do with me, or what to call what I seemed to have. I tried changing my diet, eliminating sugar and salt for a time, various allergy tests and even tried weekly allergy shots. I never really felt well, but I could not explain all that was going on and hated to complain. At one point when the pain got so bad that I could no longer work, I even was sent to a psychiatrist to see if maybe all this pain and fatigue I was feeling was "all in my head." In 1994, one doctor checked my body for a new syndrome called "fibromyalgia" (FM). "My" means muscle and "algia" means pain, which did describe my problem, but did not help me understand what was wrong. Giving what I had a name did not help any, as the various doctors and specialists could offer me no hope or treatment that was effective. I remember crying in my doctor's office begging to know if there was anything else I could do. I felt totally hopeless, suicidal, being so tired of all the pain.

Earlier that same year, I had watched my 31 year old sister die of cancer, after I gave her a bone marrow transplant that could not stop the tumors from growing back. I remember how my sister and I had many of the same symptoms that we both had lived with for years. We had simple things like numerous cold sores, the flu and colds, never ending yeast infections, eye infections, muscle pain and fatigue, depression, painful periods, allergies, and many other things that did not seem to be life threatening, as it was so common and normal in our stressful lives. We had learned to ignore our bodies hoping that if we just did not think about it, we would just get better.

I had tried MANY natural health products and vitamins and minerals for over fifteen years, but nothing really seemed to prevent my body from getting sicker and sicker. I began reading and studying about health. I had gotten to the point of unbearable pain…and could not rip paper or bear to sit down, so I could not go to work for five months. It was so scary to lose my strength and I knew after watching my sister die that maybe I should take this pain seriously as ignoring it didn't work. I even started training in a massage therapy school in search of an answer. Since the doctors could offer me no solutions, I decided I would have to look at alternative medicine. I tried a naturopath and various chiropractors. Being sick was a full time job with no pay and very costly. What I did not know at the time was that I had an autoimmune problem. Part of my pain originated inside, from my immune system attacking itself, and all the massages and adjustments in the world would not deal with the root cause. I was desperate to get better and cried out to God for an answer, praying for my immune system to be healed. I had read enough to know that was the underlying factor to my illness.

In May 96, a friend shared a strategy for health that was new to me. I felt like I had found the answer to my prayers. I knew I needed to support various systems of my body so I started on the full program of this new information. My tired, over-stressed body gained balance, strength, and energy quite quickly in comparison to how long it had taken to get so sick.

I felt this was a gift from God and a direct answer to my prayer, and I knew that my healing would take some time. I did not want to wait to tell my friends and family as I wanted healing for them now. The week before my friend Judy called to share these health principles with me, I had someone in church tell me that God was going to make a huge explosion in my life, and fill me up like a baby bird. You can imagine my excitement when Judy shared these principles with me. When I heard the various doctors speak who were training in this new field, I felt like that baby bird being fed words of life and hope.

I was so thankful when not only my body started to heal and rejuvenate, but also my spirits and my hope for living was restored. My depression lifted. Several of my friends also started on the same program and we began to heal together. It was amazing to me how in six weeks I could swim again which I had not been able to do for a few years. I noticed little things changing all the time. Then month by month I found new things would happen and I wanted to run and dance. All this energy continued to surge over time. I was gaining my memory, and clarity, like I had in high school. The "fibro-fog" was clearing all the time. Wow did I get excited!!!! I started to see the various parts of my body change and get stronger, my muscle tone increased, and I could even walk up stairs with little pain for the first time in almost fifteen years! I had fourteen of the possible trigger points that they use to diagnose FM go down to only two, much to my doctor's surprise. I could tell my whole body was gaining more health day by day in subtle ways, which to an outsider might not seem visible or important, but to me it was exciting and almost unbelievable.

At one point, about seven months into my path of recovery, I felt much worse, which was hard to accept when I had felt so good. My body started kicking out even more toxins than before, through my stool, skin rashes, with some flu like symptoms, headaches and extreme fatigue. Cold sores popped up, and canker sores, which I thought I had conquered.

Now I realize that had I continued on the comfortable path I would have not known all the places that my body needed to clean up. Yet when I was going through it, I felt confused and scared and I started to cry out to God again and pray. I remember the Lord speaking to my heart: "What do you think sick cells look like coming out?" Well that made sense, and I remember the comforting feeling of how the Lord was protecting me. Then He asked: "Whose bone marrow did you watch the cancer grow back in?" The fact that it was my own really hit me for the first time. But I had no medical proof to explain what was happening; only the sense that God was indeed protecting me. It was a knowing that all these uncomfortable symptoms were somehow for my good. Now that all my cells could communicate, they were addressing areas I never even knew I needed help in.

After three years I found an article on Medline while I was searching for Dr Dykman's study on fibromyalgia, (which I was apart of). I could barely believe my eyes when I read: "Does chronic fatigue syndrome predispose to non-Hodgkin's lymphoma?"

That is the EXACT cancer I watched claim the body of my only sister. Now it made sense medically why I seemed to have much more "correcting crisis" or detox reactions than many of my other friends who were doing what I was doing, but with very little discomfort. I learned how the greater the correcting crisis, the more thankful we should be, because the body knows before even you do what is wrong. I could see how the body's hierarchy of need worked first hand and how the toxins had to come out of my body to make room for healthy cells. I remember how it scared me when I did not understand why this was all happening.

With FM, there are so many areas that need repair. The body can only deal with so many areas at one time, and at times it can feel like you are going backwards as the repair work is going on. But slowly old injury sites healed one by one. A slipped disk in L5 felt like it had returned but was not as bad and I felt the tenderness for two weeks and then it disappeared to never again be a problem. Knees, shoulders, elbows, and ankles each became sore for days or weeks. I could see the picture in my mind of my cells doing "spring cleaning," discarding old *scar tissue that needed to be replaced with brand new healthy cells. I had clear mucus drip from my nose for almost four months. I had figured out that the more I did for my health, the worse it got, and if I cut back, the dripping stopped. This is how I learned that it was a correcting crisis, and I did not go on any allergy medications, as I normally would have done and I let nature runs its course. This helped me understand that the constant dripping was indeed good for me, even though embarrassing and uncomfortable. I noticed mucus coming out with my stool. I had a long history of problems with my ears, nose, and throat, having bronchitis many times since I was a baby. So I actually got excited when my familiar "seal" cough started with no other symptoms. I decided to do even more to speed up the process. I could see that the cough was bringing up lots of mucus with no sign of infection. It did hurt, but was really more embarrassing as I could not quit the coughing at times. It lasted for only a couple weeks. But I had realized: "How else could the bad stuff come out of my lungs?" I was not getting colds or the flu any more, so I knew my body was trying to heal.*

I went to numerous training sessions and tried to learn everything I could about preventive health. The more I learned the more confidence I had to trust my body to be doing exactly what it needed to do, regardless of how I felt. I let go of the quick fix mentality that my impatient nature wanted. I knew that in time, all the garbage would come out if I ALLOWED it to.

Now I find friends commenting on how healthy I look, and much younger than forty. It has been worth it all to get to this level of healing. Healing has been a path; not a destination and I want to keep improving. A major key was understanding how I might have to feel worse before getting better to give me the staying power to overcome my temptation to give up. Too many quit just before the healing comes as they say it costs too much and they would rather not face the uncomfortable times. I have to admit there were times I couldn't FEEL the benefits, especially when I felt worse, wondering if and when the pain would end. I think all of us wonder if something will really work for "me"— thinking that what "I have" is beyond repair. We are ALL basically just flesh and blood, with trillions of cells, and no matter what is wrong with us, it is a factor of how many of our cells are sick. So do you want to leave the toxins in your cells and see how much damage they WILL do to your whole body in time? If we leave the garbage IN our cells it is MUCH MORE PAINFUL, if not DEADLY in the long run. Following all the strategies for vibrant health and longevity helps the body communicate what needs to be worked on, cell by cell, one by one, and will in time get to all parts of the body that need repair.

DO NOT WAIT until you are sick. It costs too much in more ways than one. Neither my sister nor I thought we were going to get sick at such a young age. You cannot tell exactly what future health problems you are preventing, but with all the cancer and new autoimmune diseases, chances are your story might not be that different than mine.

I am a living example of how the body can heal and repair itself - - even when I was told there was little the doctors could do for me. I now have a vibrant, fun life, full of energy, getting to do things I had only prayed and dreamed of. I am committed to following the principles of health the rest of my life. But more amazing is that I have earned time freedom, and soon to be financial freedom. I find most of us naturally network what we believe in. I am having so much fun sharing something I love that it really does not feel like work. I had been in banking for almost twenty years and was able to leave that stressful job after only one year sharing this good news part-time. I had been looking for a better paying career for a number of years since my divorce. I am now thankful that my FM got so bad I had to quit school, as this has been a much wiser education with the bonus of making an income while I was learning. Being able to do what I enjoy, with a promising future is more of a miracle than overcoming the physical challenges. Trying to decide what to do with my life had contributed to my depression problems, as the job market looked so hopeless. Often with illness comes financial ruin, which creates a downward spiral. I am in awe of God's provision of using the bad things in my life to create an upward ladder.

I see how finding these strategies for health created a wonderful lifestyle change that has affected my well being, mentally, physically, financially, and spiritually. It has been easy to be passionate about preventive health and helping others when something really works. I hope you do not have to wait until you watch a loved one die to get serious about your own health. Start now, you are worth it!

Appendixes

{ 1 }

<u>THE AMBULANCE DOWN</u>
<u>IN THE VALLEY</u>

'Twas a dangerous cliff, as they freely confessed,
though to walk near its edge was quite pleasant,
Till over the side slipped a duke and a prince
and it had fooled many a peasant.

The people all said, something had to be done,
though their projects did not at all tally.
Some said put up a fence, 'round the edge of the cliff,
Others, an ambulance down in the valley.

A collection was made to accumulate aid,
and dwellers in highway and alley
gave dollars and cents, not to furnish a fence,
but an ambulance down in the valley.

The lament of the crowd was profound
and so loud as their hearts overflowed with great pity,
but the ambulance carried, the cry of the day
as it spread to the neighboring cities.

"For the cliff is all right if you're careful," they said,
"and if folks really trip and are falling,
It's not the slipping and sliding that hurts,
so much as the shock when they're stopping."

So for years upon years as these mishaps occurred,
quick forth would the rescuers rally,
to pick up the victims who fell from the cliff
with the ambulance down in the valley.

Said one in his plea, "It's a mystery to me
that you'd give so much greater attention
to managing effects than to addressing the cause.
Why not just work at prevention?

"The mischief, of course, should be stopped at its source.
Come friends and good neighbors, let's rally.
It makes far better sense to rely on a fence,
than on an ambulance down in the valley."

But the majority said, "He's wrong in his head.
He would end all our earnest endeavors.
He's the kind of a jerk, that would halt our good work,
but we will support it forever.

"Don't we pick them all up, just as quick as they fall
and treat them with care quite liberally?
A simple fence is of no consequence
if the ambulance works down in the valley."

Well the story is clear, as I've given it here,
though things oft' occur which are stranger,
that more humane they assert, to repair all the hurt,
than the plan of removing the danger.

Before it all ends it's time to begin
There's certainly no time to dally.
Yes, build up the fence as it makes far more sense,
than an ambulance down in the valley.

{ 2 }

UNIFIED DIETARY GUIDELINES

The President of the American Institute for Cancer Research
(AICR) commended the Unified Dietary Guidelines issued by
the American Heart Association (AHA) at its conference in New

York City on June 16, 1999.

She noted that a single set of guidelines for food choices that help prevent heart disease, stroke, diabetes, and cancer is a tremendous benefit to the public.

Beginning in 1994, AICR, in conjunction with its international affiliate, the World Cancer Research Fund (WCRF), conducted a four-year review of scientific literature on the link between diet and cancer. A panel of fifteen world-renowned scientists reviewed 4,500 studies. Their conclusions were published in the 670-page report, *Food, Nutrition and the Prevention of Cancer*, in 1997. In addition, the panel issued fourteen recommendations and six dietary guidelines based on its conclusions. Those dietary guidelines are:

1. Choose a diet rich in a **variety** of plant-based foods.

2. Eat 7 servings of vegetables and fruit daily.

3. Maintain a healthy weight and be physically **active.**

4. Drink alcohol only in moderation, if at all.

5. Select foods low in fat and salt.

6. Prepare and store food safely.

7. *And always remember* . . . Do not use tobacco in any form.

{ 3 }

REFERENCES FOR GLYCONUTRIENT STUDIES

1) Results show that two of the monosaccharides, mannose and n-acetylglucosamine, play an important role in the process of sperm and egg binding, and could be of use in some cases of infertility.

(REF) Brandelli A, Miranda PV,Tezon JG. Participation of glycosylated residues in the human sperm acrosome reaction. Possible role of N-Acetylglucosaminidase. Biochimica et

Biophysica, Acta molecular cell research. Volume 1220, number 3, 1994, 1220-1223.

2) The addition of n-acetylneuraminic (sialic) acid to rat diet improved learning and brain function; and may be of use in preventing deterioration of brain function in humans with dementia.
(REF) Carlson SE, House SG. "Oral and Intraperitoneal administration of n-acetylneuraminic acid: effect on rat cerebral and cerebellar n-acetylneuraminic acid. Journal of Nutrition 1986;986:881-886.

3) Eight monosaccharides may play a role in blocking the metastatic process in cancer (The spread of disease).
(REF) Beuth J, Ko HL, Pulverer G, Uhlenbruck G, Pichlmaier H. Presciption for Nutritional Healing. second edition. New York: Avery publishing Group, 1997

4) Research has shown that the xylose may ward off cancer and may be particularly effective against cancers of the digestive tract.
(REF) Bingham S, Williams DRR, Cole TJ, James WPT. Dietary fibre and regional large bowel cancer morbidity in Britain. *British Journal of Cancer* 1979;40:456-463.

5) Xylose infusion to rats increased lymph fluid to the heart, important in repair and immune protection of the heart.
(REF): Quiros G, Ware J. Cardiovascular and lymph flow changes caused by physiological hyperosmolar provacation in unanesthetized rats. European Surgical Research. 1984;16:69-76.

6) Researchers have discovered malabsorption and abnormal xylose absorption is associated with Multiple Sclerosis.
(REF) Gupta JK, Ingegno AP, Cook AW,Pertschuck LP. Multiple Sclerosis and malabsorption. *American Journal of Gastroenterology.* 1977;68:580-585.

7) A 1995 study revealed a fucose deficiency in patients with rheumatoid arthritis.

(REF) Kamel M, Serafi T. Fucose concentrations in Sera from patients with rheumatoid arthritis. *Clinical and Experimental Rheumatology* 1995;13:243-24.

{ 4 }
LIVING TO AGE 100 LONGEVITY TEST

(From the book, *Living to 100: Lessons in Living to Your Maximum Potential at Any Age,* by Thomas Perls, MD, Harvard Medical School)

Question 1: Do you smoke or chew tobacco, or are you around a lot of Secondhand smoke?

Cigarette smoke contains toxins that directly damage DNA and subsequently cause cancer. Cigarettes are the biggest direct source of nitrosamines humans are exposed to. These substances, along with other constituents of cigarette smoke, are potent oxidants and carcinogens that lead to accelerated aging, and diseases associated with aging.

Question 2: Do you eat more than a couple of hot dogs, slices of bacon, or a bologna sandwich a week?

Some studies suggest that 90 percent of all human cancers are environmentally induced, thirty to forty percent of these by diet. Preserved and cured meats (bacon, sausage, lunch meats, etc.) are the largest source of nitrites in our diet. Nitrites lead to the formation of nitrosoamines in our bodies, which are important environmental oxidants and carcinogens. For instance, there is a significant association between nitrosamines and stomach cancer.

Question 3: Do you cook your fish, poultry, or meat until it is charred?

Broiling can change proteins and amino acids into substances called heterocyclic amines, which are potent mutagens, or substances that can alter your DNA.

Questions 4 & 5: Do you avoid fatty foods, and emphasize fresh fruits and vegetables ?

High protein diets, and the combination of a high-fat and protein diet, have been associated with an increased risk of cancer of the breast, uterus, prostate, colon, pancreas and kidney. These foods can be inefficient sources of energy and can cause excess oxygen radical formation. Of course, saturated fats also lead to obesity and its risks (see 16 below). On the other hand, diets that emphasize fruits and vegetables have been associated with a significantly lower risk of heart disease and a better quality of life.

Question 6: Do you drink beer, wine and/or liquor in excess (more than two drinks a day)?

Excessive alcohol is a toxin that damages the liver and the mitochondria within most cells of the body. This leads to acceleration of aging and increased susceptibility to many diseases associated with aging.

Question 7: Do you drink beer, wine and/or liquor in moderate amounts (1-2 drinks a day)?

Moderate alcohol consumption has been associated with a decreased risk of heart disease. This may be one explanation for the "French paradox." The French are known for their love of high-saturated fat foods, and yet their heart disease risks may be lower (except in the cases of those who smoke cigarettes), perhaps because of the higher consumption of wine in that country.

Question 8: Do air pollution warnings occur where you live?

Numerous air pollutants are potent causes of cancer and contain oxidants that accelerate aging.

Question 9: Do you drink more than 16 ounces of coffee a day?

Excessive coffee consumption can be a sign of increased stress. Stress can lead to a hormonal imbalance that can physically stress and age numerous organs. In addition, coffee predisposes the stomach to chronic inflammation of the stomach and ulcers. Such chronic inflammation leads to the release of substances that raise the risk of heart disease. Green tea, on the other hand, has been noted for its significant antioxidant content, and tea drinkers in general appear to be healthier.

Question 10: Do you take an aspirin a day?

Eighty-one milligrams of aspirin per day has been noted to significantly decrease the risk of heart disease. This benefit may be due to the anti-blood clotting effects of aspirin. Chronic inflammation may also play a role in heart disease (see 11, below) and therefore, aspirin's effect on inflammation may also be helpful.

However, being a drug, even one aspirin a day can have serious side effects such as blindness, if used on a long-term basis. There are superior and safer ways to accomplish the same thing, such as using Omega 3 oil from flax seeds.

Question 11: Do you floss your teeth every day?

Recent scientific evidence reveals that chronic gum disease leads to the release of inflammatory and toxic substances, and certain bacteria into the blood stream. These can potentiate plaque formation in arteries and ultimately lead to heart disease. This process probably also increases the risk of stroke and accelerated aging.

Question 12: Do you have a bowel movement less than once every two days?

Keeping gut transit time under twenty hours seems to decrease the incidence of colon cancer, probably by decreasing the contact time between the gut lining and cancer-potentiating substances in the diet. These substances influence DNA damage and repair and therefore probably also influence the rate of aging as well. Epidemiological studies in humans and animal studies suggest that increasing dietary fiber will reduce the risk of certain cancers, perhaps by increasing the frequency of bowel movements.

Question 13: Do you engage in risky sexual (unprotected or promiscuous) or drug-related behavior that increase your risk of contracting HIV or viruses that can cause cancer?

Viruses such as HIV and others which are transmitted by risky behavior not only cause AIDS but also various cancers, including lymphoma. These viruses change DNA and probably, as a result, influence aging as well.

Question 14: Do you try to get a suntan?

The association between sun exposure and accelerated skin aging are clear. The ultraviolet rays in sunlight directly damage DNA. More sun means more wrinkles sooner. It also means a higher risk of deadly skin cancer. Excessive sun exposure may also have more toxic consequences for the body in general.

Question 15: Are there dangerous levels of radon in your house?

Radon is a gas emitted from various types of rock, especially granite. (New Hampshire, the Granite State, is known for its high incidence of radon exposure.) Radon is a potent carcinogen. Toxic levels of radon in the home are equivalent to smoking two packs of cigarettes a day.

Question 16: Is your weight appropriate for your height?

Obesity is associated with inefficient energy production and an increased production of oxygen radicals within cells, therefore leading to an increased risk of various cancers, heart disease and accelerated aging. It may also lead to diabetes.

Question 17: Do you live near enough to family members (other than your spouse and dependent children) whom you can drop by and visit spontaneously?

Extended family cohesiveness and frequent contact is a notable feature of centenarian families. Researchers have noted that people who do not belong to cohesive families have fewer coping resources and increased levels of social and psychological stress. Psychological stress is associated with heart disease, various cancers and increased mortality risk.

Question 18: Can you shed stress?

Centenarians shed emotional stress exceptionally well. Their stress-shedding personalities and the familial support that they receive and contribute to are important stress-reducing mechanisms.

Question 19: Does more than one member of your immediate family (parents and siblings) have diabetes?

Diabetes causes excessive exposure to glucose and therefore debilitating cross-linking of proteins. This results in age-related problems such as cataracts, impaired nerve function, eye disease, heart disease and other vascular problems.

Questions 20 & 21: What is your immediate family history?

Genetics plays a significant role in the ability to achieve extreme old age. If both sides of your family contract diseases associated with aging significantly before average life expectancy, then it behooves you to do all you can to maximize your health status. If there is extreme longevity in your family it will help significantly in your own ability to achieve good health in old age.

Question 22: Do you exercise?

Exercise leads to more efficient mitochondrial energy production and less oxygen radical formation. Exercise has been linked to lower levels of breast and prostate cancer.

Question 23: Do you take vitamin E (800 IU) and selenium (100-200 mcgm) every day?

Vitamin E is a scientifically proven antioxidant available either in the diet or as a dietary supplement. It has been shown in epidemiological studies to delay or retard the progression of Alzheimer's disease, heart disease and stroke. It also boosts the immune system. Selenium appears to have dramatic effects in preventing cancer. However, the most powerful antioxidant known is glutathione, which is most effectively raised by glyconutrients.

To take the actual test for FREE with an instant calculation of your longevity, go to: http://www.beeson.org/Livingto100/quiz.htm

{ 5 }

THE HIGH COST OF NEGLIGENCE

by Ken Anderson

"Negligence, n....2. Habitual omission of that which ought to be done, or a habit of omitting to do things, either from carelessness or design. Negligence is usually the child of sloth or laziness, and the parent of disorders in business, often of poverty."

In thirty-five years of helping and supporting people in the area of health, I have come up against some serious problems. I've seen people get over cancer, AIDS, cardiovascular disease, hepatitis, arthritis, obesity, nerve damage, etc. However, there is one condition that has been more of a challenge than all the other problems combined. It's called indifference-neglectosis.

This disease is characterized by lack of control in eating foods that are known to be harmful. A person who has this disease will eat at fast-food restaurants, buy candy bars and processed foods, drink coffee and/or carbonized beverages with tons of artificial flavors, colors, and sweeteners, and possibly even smoke cigarettes.

In the early stages, a person will have thoughts of deception, such as, "I don't eat this all the time," and, "Oh, a little won't hurt anything." Also accompanying this disease is a lack of vision for the future. Posterity is not considered. Sufferers of indifferent-neglectosis often can't see beyond their next trip to Mc Donalds, much less what their lives will be like when they are over fifty.

A person in the advanced stages of indifference-neglectosis will show even greater signs of deception. This is due to the progressive nature of the disease.

Justification of eating junk food becomes easier and more believable, therefore less necessary. Open admission of the problem accompanied by complacency is common. In extreme cases, it's no longer necessary for the person to justify or rationalize eating junk food at all.

A phenomena known as hearing-restrictitis usually accompanies indifference-neglectosis.

People with hearing restrictitis will actually experience a shrinking of the ear canal so that no sound can come through to the person, no matter how loud or how many times you warn them about their problem.

Many people, who haven't yet developed hearing-restrictitis, will ask of my counsel, sit in on one of my talks at a camp, or read books and listen to tapes, but only change for a short period of time. This phenomena, known as empty-headitis, is thought to be caused by restricted blood flow to the brain due to a very stiff neck.

Even though the hearing may be there, empty-headitis will cause the person to be a forgetful hearer rather than a faithful doer. In all cases, the person's belly, to some degree, is their god.

Although the effects of this disease can be seen at a young age, the consequences are not fully seen until the person has reached "the golden years," if they live that long. Those people who develop indifference-neglectosis can expect to live the last years of their lives in misery and pain. Many are bound to wheel chairs or are bedridden.

Most are not able to care for themselves and become burdens on their families, if their family doesn't put them into a nursing home. Medication, pain pills, frequent trips to the doctor, surgeons and operations can be expected at the end of their lives. "The golden years" become "the deathly years." A dreary, painful life awaits those who practice negligence.

Will It Be That Bad?

If you don't think so, just visit a nursing home. These people can plead ignorance because they probably did not know better, but they still suffer the consequences. 1 Corinthians 3:16-17 says, "Know ye not that ye are the temple of God, and that the Spirit of God dwelleth in you? If any man defile the temple of God, him shall God destroy; for the temple of God is holy, which temple ye are." The word "defile" in the Greek means, "to shrivel, or wither, i.e., to spoil (by any process)". I'd say that dumping junk food into your body is causing the temple to *shrivel, wither, and spoil*. Also, James 4:17 says, "Therefore to him that knoweth to do good, and doeth it not, to him it is sin."

The Wages of Sin

Blatant disregard for God's law concerning agriculture has eroded away at our land to the point that we no longer are getting adequate nutrition from what is grown on it.

In his book, <u>Overfed But Undernourished</u>, H. Curtis Wood., *Jr., M.D. stated, "The U.S. Department of Agriculture, in classifying the quality of our 415 million acres of cropland, reported that only 40 percent could be considered as satisfactory under present methods of agriculture, while 60 percent was rated as being of poor quality" (pg. 22, par. 2). That book was written in 1959! How do you think our soil rates now?*

Plants take about sixty minerals from the soil, if they are available. The fertilizer that is put back in the soil generally only has three. If the plants are taking sixty and the farmers are putting back three, do you think those other fifty-seven minerals are there anymore?

You Are What You Eat

The cells of our bodies are constantly being replaced and/or rebuilt. As these cells are being rebuilt, what are they being made from? Think of it as making a healthy cake. You throw in the ingredients: whole wheat flour, vanilla, oil, sea salt, honey, fertile eggs; but then you discover you have no eggs. The cake will not be quite right with ingredients missing. (Just imagine if white flour, processed sugar and table salt were all you had!) What inevitably happens is the body will have a craving for certain nutrients that it is not getting.

According to Dr. Erwin Gemmer, we would need to eat five times the amount of our grandparents diets in order to get the same nutrition; and even if we ate twenty times that amount, we still wouldn't get certain vital nutrients. Micah 6:14 says, *"Thou shalt eat, but not be satisfied...."* People will gorge themselves at the dinner table in an effort to feel satisfied. This produces obesity.

Naturally, people don't want to be fat, so they go on a "die-et" to try and lose weight. If they weren't getting enough nutrition when they were gorging themselves, how in the world are they going to get it if they hardly eat at all? The scary thing about those going on "die-ets" without proper supplementation, is that the body begins robbing nutrients from the bones and organs. People may experience weight loss, but it is at the expense of their bones and organs shrinking into nothing.

Lifestyle and Supplements

The way to get rid of indifference-neglectosis is to repent. Change your lifestyle to incorporate the five strategies to vibrant health and longevity. Supplements are not an option anymore. If you care about the quality of your life in the "golden years" and that of future generations, you must supplement your diet. However, you must get good supplements. Getting nutritional elements from some products is like trying to get iron from sucking on a nail or calcium from eating chalk.

As I have stated before, we also need to have a vision to be like Moses. Deuteronomy 34:7 says, *"And Moses was an hundred and twenty years old when he died: his eye was not dim, nor his natural force abated."* That's how I want the "golden years" to be for me, full of life and vigor, just like Moses. Good health is everyone's responsibility. We need to make the most of our lives, so consider your ways, and don't get indifference-neglectosis.

{ 6 }

OVERWEIGHT? CALCULATE YOUR BMI

Obesity is probably the second leading preventable cause of death in the United States after cigarette smoking, according to a professor of nutrition at the University of North Carolina.

In the largest study on over weight and mortality ever conducted, researchers looked at the medical records of more than a million Americans from 1982 through 1996 and found a clear link between being overweight and a higher risk of dying from cancer or heart disease. This study, published in the New England Journal of Medicine in October 1999, was conducted by the American Cancer Society.

In the course of the study, researchers focused on body mass index (BMI), a standard measure that factors body weight and height, and tracked participants for age and cause of death. A person's BMI should fall in the range of 19-25.

Healthy non-smoking white men, women and black men were found to have an increasing risk of death starting at a BMI of 25.

The largest white men, with a BMI of 40 or more, were found to be 2.58 times more likely to die than their healthiest peers. White women with a 40 or greater BMI were twice as likely as their healthiest counterparts to die early.

Calculate your own BMI by taking your weight in pounds, multiplied by 704.5 and then divided by your height in inches squared.

Here is an example, using my personal numbers: 157 x 704.5 = 110,606.5, divided by 4556.25 (67.75 inches times 67.75) = 24.28.

If you are not satisfied with your score, decide to do something about it right now. The most effective weight loss plan I know of (and have used myself very successfully) uses the principles in this book, including glycemic indexing and a set of safe supplements that support the natural burning of fat and at the same time increase lean muscle tissue.

{ 7 }

THE CHOLESTEROL MYTH

Cholesterol. What images come to mind when you see this word? Is it positive or negative? Is it health, or is it heart disease?

If what came to mind was negative, as something to avoid, and heart disease, then the pharmaceutical companies and food industries have been successful in getting you to believe a fabricated myth!

According to George V. Mann, M.D., professor of Medicine and Biochemistry at Vanderbilt University, *"Saturated fat and cholesterol in the diet are not the cause of coronary heart disease. That myth is the greatest scientific deception of this century, perhaps of any century."*

Russell L. Smith, Ph.D. is the author of the book, The Cholesterol Conspiracy. Dr. Smith states that *"Both the public and clinical physicians have simultaneously been swamped by an ever-growing tidal wave of exaggerations, distortions and even fabrications of the facts."*

Here's the truth. Cholesterol is good! It is a *necessary* part of every cell in your body and is essential in virtually all aspects of metabolism. Without it, we would die. That's not the impression you got from the advertisers, is it!

Cholesterol is necessary for the brain, nervous system, hormones, digestion, liver function, heart muscle contraction, calcium metabolism, bone structure and skin. Cholesterol forms 50 percent of the nervous system and serves as the conductor of nerve impulses. It is so important that your body produces four to seven times as much as you ingest and reduces its production to accommodate cholesterol intake from the food you eat.

A *deficiency* of Cholesterol results in obesity, emotional disturbances, fatigue, impotency, and many more imbalances.

How the Scam Begun

In the early 1900's, experiments were done in which rabbits were given extremely high amounts of dietary cholesterol. Their blood cholesterol rose twenty fold and a soft plaque-like disease formed on the coronary arteries. But the cholesterol levels returned to normal and the plaque disappeared when the feeding was stopped. This formed the basis of the theory that cholesterol caused coronary heart disease in humans.

Here are the flaws. The rabbits were given a synthetic form of cholesterol that easily oxidized when exposed to air (which made it toxic). Rabbits also do not metabolize cholesterol as do humans. Humans and other animals like dogs and rats do *not* develop atherosclerosis-like disease as do rabbits when given dietary cholesterol. And finally, humans do *not* develop soft plaque as did the rabbits; humans develop hard plaque which does not reverse, and it is not caused by dietary cholesterol.

Eggs and Cholesterol

One of the many foods we are warned about is eggs. In one study, seventy men were divided into three groups which ate either 3, 7, or 14 eggs a week for five months. They all had similar cholesterol levels in the beginning. The total cholesterol, LDL and HDL cholesterol and triglycerides did not change during the study for any of the groups.

An 88 year old man consumed 20-30 eggs a DAY for more than 15 years, yet maintained normal blood cholesterol levels of 150 to 200.

Cholesterol occurs only in animal foods. Yet the consumption of animal fat since 1909 actually decreased by 10 percent, whereas vegetable fat increased by over 200 percent. The increase of heart attacks has paralleled the increased use of margarine, homogenized milk and processed foods such as sugar.

According to Judith DeCava, in her book, <u>Cholesterol, Facts and Fantasies</u>, in one study, almost half of the patients had total cholesterol levels under 200, which is supposed to be safe. Yet half of this group had coronary heart disease. Of the almost 1200 who did have heart disease, one third had cholesterol levels under 200. Dr. Michael DeBakey, the famous heart surgeon, reports that 30 percent of patients who have a coronary bypass have "normal" cholesterol levels.

The Real Culprit

What IS clearly linked to heart disease is sugar. Judith DeCava, in her excellent book, <u>Cholesterol, Facts and Fantasies</u> states,

*"John Yukin analyzed the refined sugar consumed by men with atherosclerosis. The men who had heart attacks ate almost twice as much sugar as those not having heart attacks. In fact, in persons with coronary heart disease, the degree of atherosclerosis **was proportional to the amount of refined sugar consumed."** (The Lancet 1964); 2 (7349):6-8.*

As further evidence of this is the fact that the consumption of fat in the Caribbean countries is very low, but the use of sugar is very high. Cuba has one of the highest levels of sugar use, and has a higher death rate from heart attacks in men between ages 55 and 64 than the U.S.!

The Fox Guarding the Hen House

So what's perpetuating this campaign of misinformation? It's the money from the drug companies who want you to buy their cholesterol reducing drugs (that have serious side affects) and from the food industries that benefit from this scam.

Here are some examples. The American Medical Association's Executive Vice-President, Dr. James Sammons, promised physicians in 1988 of their financial rewards by stating, *"the AMA's campaign against cholesterol will bring both old and new patients to you for necessary testing, counseling and care."*

One researcher who later became a director of the National Institutes of Health bought stock in a pharmaceutical company just before announcing the results of a study favorable to the drug's effects. The editor of the AMA's publication, <u>Circulation</u>, also received stock options on the same drug company.

Jane Heimlich began doing extensive research on this cholesterol issue in 1989. In her book, <u>What Your Doctor Won't Tell You</u>, she concludes,

"There is no question that the cholesterol program…benefits three powerful groups in our society to the tune of billions of dollars. These three are the medical profession, the pharmaceutical industry, and the food companies."

{ 8 }

<u>CONSPIRACY AGAINST OUR CHILDREN</u>

By Dr. Erwin Gemmer

Dr. Erwin Gemmer is a health practitioner with over 25 years of experience. He has attended to over 400,000 patient visits. He has spoken to more than 1200 audiences on health, and over 1,000,000 people have heard his "Who Stole America's Health" message.

Americans would be horrified if they picked up today's newspaper and it said that 2,500,000 children across the nation were being given cocaine by their parents and doctors to make them behave better. Unfortunately, this is so close to what is in fact happening that it takes a chemist to tell the difference. Millions of children, and most of them are boys, are being dosed with mind-altering, highly addictive stimulants that work on the brain much like cocaine does. The drug is methyl-phenidate hydrochloride. Most of us know it by the trade name Ritalin. Its use has shot up 600% in less than ten years. We are now hearing reports of elementary schools where 40%, and even 50%, of the students are taking Ritalin daily on a prescription basis.

How can this be? Simply put, a giant pharmaceutical company, a person of the psychiatric industry, and certain branches of the education establishment have teamed up and are pushing to convince people that Ritalin is good and is safe. Well-meaning parents, as well as school nurses and principals, often do not know that other solutions are readily available, so they finally bend under the pressure and begin supporting the practice of medicating the kids. The drug is supposed to help kids sit still, listen, and perhaps focus better, but even if its use did consistently provide these benefits, which it doesn't, what are we teaching these students in the process? These young students who are given the drug, and all the other students looking on, are getting a very clear message: *Take drugs when faced with a challenge. Take drugs to perform better. Take drugs to fit in and be like everyone else.* And, even though there is a constant effort in most communities to tell kids to stay away from drugs, our actions are speaking so much louder than our words.

Ritalin is not an innocent little pill like we have been led to believe. Studies cited by the Drug Enforcement Agency have shown that Ritalin and cocaine cause nearly identical reactions in the very same brain cells. Tests have also shown that cocaine addicts can hardly tell the difference between the two, and Ritalin abuse is now generating more Emergency Room visits among certain age groups than cocaine. In several states, lawsuits have been filed against school officials and doctors, alleging malpractice and fraud specifically because the parents involved had not been advised of Ritalin's severe side effects.

You see, Ritalin often gives the appearance of helping, but there are consequences. Many kids become plagued with nervousness, insomnia, weight loss, stunted growth, depression, dizziness, nausea, headaches, drowsiness, chest pains, rapid or irregular heart beat and many other problems too numerous to list here. Then when Ritalin's use is finally discontinued, withdrawal symptoms can appear such as long-term depression and thoughts of suicide.

Reports from another study even state that long-term use may cause a wasting away of the cerebral cortex, that is, the part of the brain needed for higher levels of thought. With all this data available, to me it is absolutely criminal that Ritalin prescriptions are written so indiscriminately. I was shocked when I first learned the criteria used to rationalize placing a child on Ritalin. There are no laboratory tests, no brain scan, no x-rays, no measurements. Nothing even vaguely scientific to demonstrate the existence of a medical disease that may need to be treated with a drug. Instead, the American Psychiatric Association circulates a publication called *The Diagnostic and Statistical Manual of Mental Disorders*. In it are lists of things to watch for in a child to supposedly determine if that child has an attention disorder.

Now I want you to remember back to when you were in school, and think of how many of the smartest, most creative kids in your class, maybe you included, would have been told that they had a mental disorder if this bogus diagnostic method had been in use then. This is the list that has put the majority of almost three million grade-school- aged kids on Ritalin:

1. Does the child often fidget with his hands or feet, or squirm in his seat?
2. Have difficulty remaining seated when asked to do so?
3. Run about or climb in situations in which it is inappropriate?
4. Have difficulty playing quietly?
5. Does the child often blurt out answers before questions have been completed?
6. Have difficulty sustaining his attention?
7. Talk excessively?
8. Shift from one uncompleted activity to another?
9. Not seem to pay attention when spoken to directly?
10. Does the child often make mistakes in schoolwork?
11. Have difficulty waiting his turns in games or group activities, or get easily distracted?

There they are. If the answer is Yes to some of these, that's all the evidence that's needed to drug the child. Can you believe that? Through this, almost 3,000,000 kids have been put on a drug similar to cocaine, for being kids. According to the International Narcotics Board, that is almost 12% of all the boys in this country, aged six through 14; plus hundreds of thousands of girls. You see, there is hardly a boy alive, and very few girls, who couldn't be labeled with a disorder when using this list as the gauge.

Even Albert Einstein, if he had been born in the last decade or so would have perfectly fit the profile of someone having attention deficit and supposedly needing Ritalin. He didn't speak until he was seven. His teacher described him as mentally slow, unsociable, and adrift in his foolish dreams. You can rest assured that today, there would have been an all-out effort to have him medicated. And he certainly wouldn't have been alone. In school, Thomas Edison's thoughts often wandered, and his body was perpetually moving in his seat. His teacher said that he was unruly and too stupid to learn anything. Hard to believe now considering they were talking about the guy whose research later gave the world light bulbs, tape recorders, and hundreds of other inventions.

Walt Disney had several of the characteristics used to diagnose ADHD, as did Alexander Graham Bell, Leonardo da Vinci, Mozart, Henry Ford, Benjamin Franklin, Abraham Lincoln, the Wright Brothers, and the list goes on. Their accomplishments speak for themselves, yet every one of these great minds and thousand of others like them would probably have been labeled with a mental disorder and put on Ritalin if they had gone to grade school in America today. Fortunately for them, and for us, they missed being drugged but what about our children? Do we want to stunt their initiative and creativity by drugging them? Wouldn't it be wiser instead to find out what is really stopping each of these young people from doing their very best at school?

Medicating kids with Ritalin does not correctly address a single one of these challenges. Would we allow millions of babies to be drugged every time they cried instead of attending to their basic needs? If not, tell me why are we allowing millions of children — our future, our greatest national asset — to be drugged month after month simply for being kids?

It is often explained to parents that their kids have an alleged chemical imbalance which is causing hyperactivity, and that Ritalin will level off this imbalance; but what they aren't told is that not one shred of scientific evidence has ever demonstrated that such an imbalance exists. Nor are they told that the Ritalin they are being offered as the solution to this imaginary problem is a type of Speed.

Another story that parents are told is that their child is only receiving a low dose of Ritalin. "So don't worry, it's no problem," they say. But would we buy into that story if they were saying, "We want to put your child on heroin, but don't worry, it's just a low dose of heroin."? When a policeman catches somebody with cocaine, does he say, "Oh, you're just using a little bit of cocaine today, no problem. Sorry to bother you. Would you like a donut to go with it?" Or, does the user get hauled off to jail?

Listen, there are better ways. Here are a few examples of actions we could start taking right now to change things for the better: First, reduce the amount of time children spend each day watching television and playing video games. Beyond a shadow of a doubt, when kids spend too much time with these electronic devices, they definitely do worse in school. So limit their use in the evening. Shut them off in time for the kids to get a good night's sleep; and make it a rule, no TV, no video games before school in the morning, *ever!*

Second, encourage kids, stop being critical, and instead catch them doing things right, praise them, and let them know they're noticed. Truly listen to your children when they are talking and let them know you really care and constantly remember the bumper sticker that says, "Hugs, not drugs."

The main thing for all of us to remember is this: if a child is having trouble applying himself to his studies, there are reasons. The symptoms that children exhibit are always cries for help, and as responsible adults we need to look behind the symptoms for the actual roots of the problem. Many of today's most exciting discoveries that are helping children are being made within the field of nutrition. This probably doesn't come totally as a surprise to you since after all, most of us have observed how virtually any child can be made hyperactive and unteachable if fed enough sweets; and conversely, when white sugar, candy, and sugary breakfast cereals are reduced, behavioral improvements are often almost immediate. But there is much more besides the overuse of sugar to be said about today's nutritional challenges.

Scientists are now seeing that all sorts of foods lack nutrients that they once had, and many of them believe that this is contributing to learning difficulties and many other childhood problems.

Glyconutritionals are a special type of carbohydrates that are essential for our well being yet are almost totally absent in our modern-day food. The discovery of these glyconutritionals and what they can do in our bodies is so exciting and revolutionary that the scientists involved earned the top biochemistry discovery of the year 1994 award from the American Naturopathic Medical Association.

These glyconutrients can give all the adults and children who consume them a greater chance to function at their best, both physically and mentally; and I believe we'll find that many of the symptoms referred to earlier might be related to shortages of these key nutrients, and that appropriate standardized nutraceutical supplements could be our best bet at over-coming these challenges.

With their use, more and more kids might be free from dangerous medications, and this could reduce the incidence of bizarre drug reactions like six-year-old Mardie from Florida, who cried uncontrollably while on Ritalin; like five-year-old Tim from Indiana who began having hallucinations and jumped at his mother screaming, "The bugs are going to get me!" (he told his mother that hundreds of bugs were falling from the ceiling); Or like ten-year-old Melvin from Georgia who attempted suicide after taking the drug.

Other countries are banning this drug entirely. It is time for this disgusting experiment to come to an end here also.

The drug promoters are even pressing for legislation that would allow Ritalin and other drugs to be given to our children without parental consent through the clinics they want placed in each of our schools. It is a national disgrace already, but it is going to get a lot worse if we don't act fast, and as bad as Ritalin is, it is only part of the monster.

Unfortunately, on top of all these drugs, other depraved forces have insidiously been at work in the schools too. Specifically, years ago a thrust was started to lead educators as far as possible away from traditional values; educators who would later pass these removal-of-values teachings on down to our children. Here's what I mean. At the risk of raising your blood pressure a bit, listen to this: addressing the 1973 Childhood International Education Seminar, psychiatrist Chester Pierce stated and I quote: *"Every child in America entering school at the age of five, is mentally ill because he comes to school with certain allegiances to our founding fathers, towards our elected officials, towards his parents, towards a belief in a supernatural being. It is up to you as teachers to make all these sick children well."*

Now most teachers don't agree with this line of thinking, but a lot of the books and classes seem to be pointing kids in that direction anyhow. And nothing could help more to achieve these perverted goals than to deaden the children's minds with narcotic drugs. Unless we stop it fast, our country is about to lose a whole generation to prescription mind-altering drugs, and the pharmaceutical companies will profit raking in billions of dollars as children become addicted by the millions now, and remain hooked in varying degrees throughout their adult life.

People, we are faced with a classic David vs. Goliath situation here. It is not easy to start turning a mess like this around, but we have no choice. We have to stop this drugging of the children. It is the responsibility of every person who hears this message, to do what he/she can now. Keep your own children free from mind-altering drugs. Speak out against the misuse of these drugs and help get this message into every home in America. If whole countries around the world can have high academic achievement without giving their students Ritalin, then why not us? It is time to replace this insanity with common sense so that our children can again be bright, creative, happy and interested in learning.

Remember, Ritalin is a narcotic, a highly addictive stimulant classified by the Food and Drug Administration under Schedule 2 of the Controlled Substances Act. Included in this category are cocaine, opium, and morphine. And as with these other drugs, an adult possessing Ritalin without a prescription could go to jail. Isn't it time for us to quit forcing this dangerous substance onto our six-, eight-, and ten-year-olds?

*This transcription is an edited version of Doctor Gemmer's excellent cassette, "Conspiracy Against Our Children." For a **free** copy of this shocking tape, call (800) 700-1238.*

{ 9 }

My Personal Journey Back to Health:

I had turned totally blue, and my young mother didn't know what to do. Fortunately, my grandmother did, and I was rushed to the hospital. At a fragile age of 6 months, I had had an allergic reaction to milk that almost killed me.

In the third grade, a boy, thinking I was cheating at a game of "Prison Ball," pushed me down and kicked me in the back, which began 37 years of chronic back pain and instability.

Later in grade school, I was tested and found to have allergies to 14 types of grasses and to dust and certain foods. I suffered with hay fever practically year round. I took allergy medication twice a day for 14 years, including one year of weekly shots, with little relief. I would frequently take two handkerchiefs to school, and not have them be enough to handle my runny nose.

In high school, I started having episodes of tachycardia for several minutes at a time; my heart would race at 200 beats per minute. This continued for about 30 years.

I developed chronic nervous habits, stuttering and nervous twitches with my face which continued for over 30 years.

In 1976, I was diagnosed with the beginning stage of arthritis in my neck.

In 1984, I developed a cataract in my left eye. That same year, my back pain was further aggravated by a fall that resulted in a back fracture that partially paralyzed the lower half of my body for a time. The doctor informed me that I would continue to be at risk of my spinal cord being pinched off and having permanent paralysis from my waist down.

I was diagnosed with a heart murmur and an abnormal EKG. In 1988 a life insurance application was declined due to a high white blood cell count, which was initially suspected to be from an HIV infection (it was not).

I was about 25-30 pounds overweight, and the stress from a second failed marriage was contributing to very poor digestion as well as fleeting suicidal thoughts. I also had developed such a severe irregular heart beat that it was sometimes even disrupting my conversations due to the severe coughing that would occur when I talked.

In 1993, I began to realize that I was having serious trouble remembering phone numbers and other important details. Psoriasis was showing up on my elbows, and frequently my skin would crack between my toes and on my lower lip. I had chronic rashes that itched in various unmentionable areas of my body. The toll of stress was showing up all through out my body and mind.

Between 1994 and 1996, I began implementing all five strategies to vibrant health, happiness and longevity as described in this book, including the essential nutrients. Now at almost a half a century old, I look like I'm 35, feel like I'm 25, and I have a sense of being fully alive.

At slightly under 5'8," my waist is now 34 inches and my weight is 157 pounds, which is the lowest I've weighed in 30 years. My percentage of body fat as measured by underwater testing is under 14 percent, which puts me as having less body fat than 92 percent of men my age. I now look slim and vibrant, and no longer struggle with my weight as I had for the last thirty years. I have no back or neck pain, no allergies or hay fever, no tachycardia, no irregular heart beat and no detectable heart murmur. I have a normal EKG, healthy skin, an above average vital capacity (lungs), a phenomenal memory, mental acuity and feel great and happy all the time. My resting pulse rate is an "athletic" 45-50. I exercise at a pulse rate of 140-150 without being out of breath (I can still have a normal conversation). I can do 100 pushups. My blood pressure is 110 over 75 and my cholesterol levels are better than normal. I have high energy and stamina, and fully expect to live a healthy active life well past 100.

I practice what I preach by faithfully following all five of the strategies that I advocate. The supplements I use that are a critical factor in my excellent health are listed in the order of importance to me.

1. Glyconutrient complex for immune support and modulation
2. Phytonutrient blend for antioxidant support
3. Plant sterols (dioscorea) for hormonal support and energy
   (an alternative to these first three items is a whole food protein bar designed to be a delivery system for glyconutrients, phytonutrients and plant sterols)
4. Vitamin, mineral and anti-oxidant complex (in a food matrix for superior assimilation and absorption)
5. Flax seed or flax seed oil
6. Psyllium seed husks for additional fiber or an advanced intestinal health support product
7. Advanced Master Mineral Complex
8. Hydrochloric Acid and digestive enzymes
9. Vitamin C
10. Lecithin

I consider the first five items the most critical and important supplements I could use to support my vibrant health and longevity. The first three are considered as a basic optimal health plan.

Almost every morning, after exercising, I make a delicious protein drink for breakfast (using a Vita-Mix or blender). I put in three raw eggs (some people have concerns about using raw eggs), soy milk, two or three tablespoons of flax seeds, a tablespoon of lecithin, protein powder (certified as low glycemic by the Glycemic Research Institute), frozen blueberries, strawberries, a small amount of frozen banana and usually some Tofu and flax seed oil (optional). It tastes great, makes me feel great and helps me to stay looking great.

{ 10 }

DISCOVERING *TREASURE* IN TROUBLES AND *STRENGTH* IN STRUGGLES

One of the most common perspectives that people hold is that a negative personal history precludes and *disqualifies* them from having a powerful future. This perspective is not only very limiting, it is very disabling and disempowering. It can prevent you from even *trying* to make a better life and future.

History, however, clearly indicates the exact opposite: problems, troubles, struggles, disappointments and "failures" can be the most powerful *preparation* for a meaningful life of significant impact and contribution. Without the stress and challenges of struggle and problems, we would not need to grow and become stronger. We would miss much more of our potential than we already do.

For example, if you ease the struggle of a butterfly by helping it out of its cocoon, you will have disabled it from being able to fly. A life of ease breeds weakness. For example, scientists discovered that without the constant stress of gravity, bones give up "unneeded" calcium and within a few days, we would lack the strength to walk, as evidenced by astronauts returning from space.

Instead of appreciating the benefits that we can *only* get from struggle and challenge, we frequently hold a perspective of resentment that disempowers us and stunts our growth.

Why Me?

We often ask the futile question, "*Why* did this happen to me?"

It may be that the problem was exactly what you needed for your next stage of personal growth. Instead of believing that there must be a *benefit* in this situation, either now or in the future, we look at the immediate *inconvenience*. Here are a few of the unavoidable consequences of this unhealthy, but all too common, perspective.

Anxiety or anger over our problems creates an unhealthy psychological stress that weakens our immune systems. This leaves us more susceptible to illness, including cancer and other common degenerative diseases.

Resenting the challenge also robs us of the happiness that could have been ours, even during the struggle.

And then it gets worse. Because we influence others, our anxiety or anger creates stress for *them* and pulls them down as well, robbing *them* of joy that they could have had. So, not only have we ripped ourselves off, we have ripped off someone else too. And it may not end there.

The Infection Spreads

The negative influence we have on other people can spread like an infection. And they, in turn, can spread it to others, sometimes amplifying the negative effect through each generation because it is combined with existing anxiety and/or anger on unrelated issues.

In essence, there can be a snowball effect – and the "straw that broke the camel's back" effect. Without having a clue, we can contribute to the unhappiness of dozens or hundreds of people, while we ignorantly think that it is just *our* problem.

Forfeiting our Future

Another crippling effect this limited perspective often has is that it robs us of more than the happiness in the present—it will insidiously rob us of our future happiness as well! We feel unqualified and perhaps *disqualified* to attempt something great, based on how we interpret our past or current problems, failures and struggles.

If you feel like a loser, why would you even *try* something new? You think that you've *already* had enough disappointment and pain from failure, and you certainly don't need any more.

A different perspective could be that *because of* all your past and current disappointment and pain, you are better *prepared* than ever to do something new and different, or even great! With the accumulation of all that experience and education from the School of Hard Knocks, you are positioned to really do something significant.

Plus, you can look at it from this perspective as well: "I've had enough—I'm not going to live this way any more!" This perspective (attitude) can powerfully propel you into a fantastic fulfilling future. Instead of caving in under the pressure, *harness* the pressure to propel yourself into your exciting future toward your destiny.

It's your choice. You can take the negativity from your past and allow it to explode like gasoline in your face, to cripple or destroy you, or you can take that same negativity and use it as fuel to drive your vehicle to success.

My Story is Mostly Negative

The best example I can give you is my own life. I wanted you to know some of the negativity of my past, so that you can clearly see two things.

First, it is possible that you, too, can have a great future — even if your past has been quite negative.

Second, your negative past, though it is full of struggle, disappointments and "failures," inevitably has an undiscovered significant value to you in terms of *preparing* you for a great destiny. But this benefit is not automatic—it depends upon you shifting your perspective to a positive and expectant outlook.

I was born on Christmas Eve in 1951 — with a major disadvantage. Three months earlier, my father, who had just graduated from Bible school, died from a ruptured appendix. The doctor had misdiagnosed his illness as food poisoning.

I never met my biological father; instead I started off with a heartbroken and grieving mother. Probably due to the stress of this situation, I had a severe allergy to milk. On one occasion this allergy made me turn blue. If my grandmother had not recognized the severity of my condition and rushed me to the hospital, I would have died.

Before I was two years old, my mother remarried. This man was not well-equipped emotionally to be my stepfather, having never recovered from trauma he had suffered in the war. He was quite abusive, both verbally and physically. It seemed that his favorite words were stupid, idiot or crazy.

I lived in Gresham, Oregon, my first eighteen years, dreaming about the day I would finish high school and escape the terror.

Predictably, I grew up feeling very insecure. I was introverted and shy (I am still an introvert). I had a problem with stuttering. I lacked the basic social skills to even have friends.

To compensate for these problems, I tried sports, including wrestling, swimming, football, baseball and track. I dropped out of the football, baseball and track, and never got any better than average in wrestling or swimming.

My Compensating Backfires

My first year in high school, I discovered that I could get high grades. I started reading a lot, and developed my analytical mind. In fact, I overcompensated by becoming excessively analytical and a very judgmental self-righteous "Pharisee".

I had successfully turned my good gift of intellect into a social handicap.

This arrogant mindset continued to be a painful blind spot for many years. It still continues to resurface, and I deal with it.

I had decided I wanted to get a Ph.D. in nuclear physics. But just before I graduated, I decided that I wanted to first go to a Bible college in Grand Rapids, Michigan, for one or two years to get a good foundation for my life. However, after only a couple months, in the fall of 1970, I decided that people were more important than science (as fascinating as science was to me) and chose to stay the full five years and major in Bible and Theology.

My First Job Failure

I vividly remember my first sales job. It was the summer of 1972. I was recruited by Southwestern Books to sell Bible storybooks door-to-door for the summer. I didn't have any confidence that I could do such a thing, but they convinced me that they would fully train me, and I could earn up to $5,000 for the summer.

A week after I was married, we went to Nashville for a week of training. Then they sent us to Long Beach, California, for the summer. It was a good growing experience, and at least I didn't quit. But at the end of the summer I had no money and owed the company $500!

In 1973 I discovered how to overcome my severe allergies and hay fever with nutrition. This launched me into an intensive self-study of health and nutrition that has continued to this present day. I received some specialized advanced training by a number of progressive medical and holistic alternative type doctors from 1978 to 1999, and even worked as an unlicensed holistic health doctor for a number of years and taught classes. Though I had some great success helping people, it seldom gave me sufficient income.

More Disappointment

After graduating from college in 1975, I spent five disappointing years as an intern at a small church in Anaheim, California.

During this time, I discovered network marketing. I was

intrigued by the concepts of multiplication and leverage and the dream of financial freedom. This marked the beginning of nineteen years of frustration and failure as I went through forty or fifty companies with very little success. This included buying $5,000 of water filters that collected dust in the garage for years.

During this same period, I gained some experience in life insurance, and for a few years did fairly well. In 1980, after building a good-sized organization, my manager decided that I was not competent to manage my organization and took away my people against my will. During this period, I had my car repossessed. I ended up quitting.

I started my own janitorial business and did most of the work myself. Within two years that fizzled and failed.

Marital Disappointments

In 1982, I experienced the harsh devastation of divorce and lost my house to foreclosure.

I then met a lady from San Diego. We fell in love, and became engaged. She refused to marry me until I had a steady income, which never happened. Three years later, through a lot of pain and disappointment, that relationship failed.

Later that year I met someone else and married for the second time. What followed were seven painful years of "hell." Because it was so bad, both of my sons moved out; one to live with my mother in Oregon and the other to live with my brother in Washington. I was failing as a father too.

In 1990 I moved to Washington and attempted to sell insurance again. I was not successful. Other companies I worked with went out of business without paying what was owed me.

In 1993, I went through my second divorce. I now felt doubly disqualified from life, since I believe marriage is supposed to be permanent. At the same time, it was a huge relief.

At the End of My Rope

At this point, I had no job, no place of my own to live and owed over $25,000 on credit cards (and I was six months behind on payments). I owed far more than that in personal debt.

In desperation, I asked a neighbor if my son and I could stay in his basement for a few weeks. He graciously consented. After six months, he insisted that we leave.

I then met a family who had an empty unfinished basement. I asked if I could stay for a few weeks. It turned out I stayed a year. Initially I was unable to even pay the $200 rent or afford my own food.

New Hope

In February of 1994, I got a call from someone (Jett) who had been given my name by someone else (Ray Robbins) I had known from another failed MLM venture. Jett convinced me that this new company was different. I decided it was either too good to be true or too good to miss.

Fortunately, I took my new business seriously. I borrowed money to fly to Dallas to see the company. Then, because I felt I needed to invest in my new business by having plenty of product on hand, I did one of those last resort desperate kind of things—I called my mother. I hoped she had a credit card that she could use to give me a cash advance of $1,900. I promised to pay her back within thirty days plus all the fees and interest.

She said no. After going back and forth several times, I finally convinced her to take a chance on me. I was able to sell enough product to pay her back in thirty days as I had promised.

Seven weeks after starting, I got my first check from the company, Mannatech. It was for $7. After working eighty hours a week for seven weeks, I had earned only about one cent per hour!

I was discouraged, but I still had enough faith to keep going. One week later, on April 7, my car was repossessed. Since 99 percent of my time was spent on the phone, it didn't slow me down much.

Forty days later, with some help, I was able to get it back. My monthly income with Mannatech continued to increase. By my seventh month, my income had reached over $10,000 for that month, which was more than I had made in my entire life in network marketing. By the end of the year, it had exceeded $20,000 per month.

Now my income is more in a month than most people earn in two years. We own a beautiful home on Lake Sammamish, with a dock, ski boat and Sea Doo. I bought my wife a new gold LS 400 Lexis (owned free and clear) and I drive a Lexus RX 300. More importantly, I fully enjoy my freedom. But the greatest blessing by far has been my marriage to Diana on May 7, 1995. We are free to enjoy life and do what we feel is most important, which is to serve God and help people.

What was Different This Time

As to why I was blessed with such great success as fast as it occurred (which is not typical) is primarily due, I believe, to God's grace. It certainly helped having phenomenal products with a fantastic compensation plan and great leadership in the company.

The other strategic factor was this: I was ready. I had been learning and growing through all the struggles and disappointments over the years. I was being prepared because I used my faith to maintain a healthy perspective on life. I continued to believe that someday things would work out for the best, as long as I never quit praying. I had been feeding my faith and positive perspective by attending seminars, reading self-improvement books including the Bible and listening to self-development tapes for years (such as Jim Rohn and Zig Ziglar).

It is always better to be prepared without a good opportunity than to have a good opportunity without being prepared.

Dangerous Assumptions

So why do people tend to get stuck in an unhealthy and negative perspective? It often is due to the common thinking (assumption) that our future will be a *continuation* of our past.

It's like expecting a rolling ball to continue in the same direction. People often act like a mindless ball—they just keep doing what they have always done, because they know nothing else, and thus expect nothing different.

Because we do have a mind, unlike an unconscious rolling ball, we have the power of choice. We have the power (and responsibility) to choose our direction and our destiny. We are not victims of fate. The ball is unconscious, so it has no choice. Unless we choose to be conscious, we too, like the unconscious ball, will be unable to change our direction or our life. How tragic! How sad!

Does a Dog Love Bones?

Here's another example. Consider this: Does a dog love bones? Most people would say. "Yes, of course." That is certainly one perspective.

I say dogs don't particularly like bones. Actually they *settle* for bones. The proof of this is in giving the dog a choice between steak and bones. About what percentage of the time do you think the dog will choose a bone over the steak? Pretty close to zero!

So, the dogs appear to love bones because they don't normally have a choice. The reality is that dogs settle for bones.

What Are You Settling For?

What are you settling for? Are you settling for "bones"? If so, it is because you don't realize that you have a choice. Perhaps you are holding onto a disempowering interpretation of life that says that you are *disqualified* from being able to choose "steak" because of your negative or abusive past. This may also show up as feeling undeserving or unable.

You have the power to use the rough rocks from your past to build walls and prisons, or to build steps to your future, or even better, to build a palace instead of a prison.

And this is best done with happiness and gratitude, and acknowledging that you are better prepared *because of your past.*

Why Share Your "Failures"?

There is also a huge benefit (of which you may be unaware) that comes from *sharing* the story of your negative past, with all its disappointments and failures. When you share your negative past, people tend to identify with parts of your history (since they too have bad stuff happen to them). The result of this is twofold.

First, people will feel more secure and comfortable around you, since they realize that you are not different from them. Instead of seeing you as a possible threat, they will be open to new ideas, and begin to think that if you can do it, so can they.

Second, people are more likely to respect and trust you, since you had the courage to be open and authentic. In this position, you are better able to help them make a positive decision since they will be less defensive.

If you are willing to adopt a different perspective, you can discover buried treasure in your troubles and strength in your struggles.

Empowered with this perspective, you can rejoice instead of resent. Empowered with this perspective, you can have victory instead of being a victim. Empowered with this perspective, instead of living with frustration, fear and failure, you can live with fascination, faith and a fantastic future.

What's Really at Stake

There is too much at stake here. If you interpret your past as disabling, you have chosen to mentally cripple yourself. As a self-created handicapped person, you will never be able to influence and inspire lives or achieve anything great. Not only will you be the loser and miss your destiny, so will the thousands of people who you deprived of your powerful influence (both directly and indirectly).

Instead, embrace a positive perspective. Your destiny and others is at stake! It's your choice! Fear or faith! I invite and challenge you to choose the road less traveled.

The Power of YOUR Story

One of the most personally empowering things you can do is to write out your "life story." Even if you never show it to anyone, it can be extremely healing and insightful. But its greatest value is when you share it with others. Your story can be easily printed in a small tract that you can just give to people. Why would you want to do this?

Many people are doing this in order to more effectively share their personal experience with God and how He has changed their lives. Your personal story and how God has been part of your life can be one of the most powerful tools you have to influence, help and impact the lives of others. It gives you a very powerful way to make a difference.

Jerry Brandt, a close friend of mine, has created a fantastic workshop (an audio tape album with a detailed workbook) that can help you write your story and get it printed in a small four-by-five inch (folded) tract with your picture on the front. Plus you'll learn effective ways to share it.

Having your story printed in a personalized tract makes it easy and exciting to share it with others. Having your story in a printed tract also can greatly increase your influence and ability to help others find God. If you are at all interested, contact "Just Ask Me" with Jerry Brandt at jbrandt4him@hotmail.com or (877) 771-1319. A free sample can be sent to you.

I strongly encourage you to empower your life by writing and printing your story, and then share it with everyone you meet.

{ 11 }
FOUNTAIN OF YOUTH MOVEMENTS

I have found that these five patterns of movement energize me instantly, as well as reduce my stress. They are claimed to reverse the aging process, and I believe they do, as I have been doing them myself for two years. As such, I refer to them as the Fountain of Youth movements. I believe the reason they work so well for people is because they reduce stress and support the immune system function. They are based on a fictional story in the book, *"Ancient Secret of the Fountain of Youth"* by Peter Kelder.

Thousands of people, including myself use them daily. I recommend that you do too, as part of your personal health and wellness plan. Your investment of time is only a short three to five minutes, but your payoff can be tremendous and very long-term.

Here is what Lucy Beal says about the "Fountain of Youth" movements: *"They actually cause circulation into all of the body's glands and organs, such as the thyroid, adrenals, etc. They tone the region from the jaw line to the upper hip the most so that people get their tummies flat, their upper arms toned and the women love that their double chins go away and they can zip up their pants, cause their waists to get thinner. They are the easiest, laziest way I have found to tone up. So I have done them for years. It's sort of like a cup of coffee in the morning without the coffee."*

"Since I started doing these five movements, my insomnia and eczema disappeared completely (I'm 53). After 25 years of bifocals, I no longer need glasses. I feel like I'm 16 again, but I'm really going to miss my lovely silver hair. It's the only thing I like about being older." Ida Schultz, Salt Lake City, Utah.

"With these five movements, I am building muscle and dropping fatty tissue. I feel much better now." Charles Knower, California

"My memory was getting so bad I was ashamed. Now, after using these for two months, I seem to be getting clarity of mind, and much, much more energy. My friends notice the change too. I am truly thankful

that at age 62 I am "youthing" instead of aging." Adeline Neveu, Yakima, Washington.

Fountain Of Youth Movement #1

Before I start, I take a couple minutes to lay on the floor and stretch all my muscles in every direction I can.

The first Fountain of Youth movement consists of merely spinning around in a clockwise direction (moving from left to right) with your arms outstretched to the side for seven to twenty-one times. Start by doing three to no more than seven rotations. Each day, increase this by two until you are able to easily do twenty-one at a time. This is the most you need to do at one time. I experience an immediate reduction of stress and an energizing effect with just this first one. If you do not have time to do all five movements at least do this one every morning.

Fountain Of Youth Movement #2

The second Fountain of Youth movement consists of lying flat on the floor on your back. Bend your chin down onto your chest and at the same time, while keeping your knees straight, lift both of your legs up until they are straight up, or as close as you can get to straight up. Resume the original position. This is one cycle. Repeat this cycle as many times as is comfortable up to seven times. Make sure you keep breathing. Each day, increase the number of repetitions by two until you can do twenty-one. This was the most difficult one for me initially. I could only do one or two at first, and it was a strain on my lower back. Eventually, I could easily do twenty-one, and now I have no more back pain at all.

Fountain Of Youth Movement #3

The third Fountain of Youth movement consists of kneeling on the floor with your body erect. Bend your head forward and touch your chin to your chest, or as close as you can get comfortably. Then reverse the direction and gently arch your head and back as far back as you comfortably can. This is one cycle. Repeat this cycle as many times as is comfortable up to seven times. Breathe in deeply as you arch your spine, and breathe out as you return to the erect position. Each day, increase the number of repetitions by two until you can do twenty-one.

Fountain Of Youth Movement #4

The fourth Fountain of Youth movement consists of sitting on the floor with your legs straight in front of you with your feet 12 inches apart, your knees straight and your palms flat on the floor next to your thighs. Bend your chin down onto your chest. Now lift your body up so that your torso is parallel to the floor as you bend your head back. At this point, your body should resemble a table. Now tense all your muscles in your body. Finally, relax your muscles as you return to the original sitting position, and rest before repeating the procedure. Breathe in as you raise up, hold your breath as you tense the muscles, breathe out completely as you come down. Continue breathing in the same rhythm as long as you rest between repetitions. Repeat this cycle as many times as is comfortable up to seven times. Make sure you keep breathing. Each day, increase the number of repetitions by two until you can do twenty-one.

Fountain Of Youth Movement #5

The final Fountain of Youth movement consists of lying on the floor in a pushup position with your arms straight and your hands placed in front of you somewhat wider than your shoulders. Your elbows will be locked the entire time. Spread your feet fairly wide, with your knees touching the floor. Lift your head up toward the ceiling. This is your starting position, with your back now arched.

Now lift your body by reversing the position of your back, so your buttocks are as high as you can lift it. As you do this, bend your chin down onto your chest. Now you will look somewhat like a tent. Return to the original position. This is one cycle. Repeat this cycle as many times as is comfortable up to seven times. Breathe in deeply as you raise your body and breathe out fully as you lower it. Each day, increase the number of repetitions by two until you can do twenty-one.

As you do each of these movements, think of your health goals, and someone you appreciate.

{ 12 }
TEN-SECOND STRESS RELIEF

Some of the most useful and practical tools I've discovered for enhancing my health and the health of others is from applied kinesiology, which came out of chiropractic health care. I've been involved with Touch For Health and kinesiology since 1978, and am a certified instructor and a professional health provider. I've been trained by some of the best doctors and teachers, including Bruce Dewe, M.D., from New Zealand; John Diamond, M.D., from Australia; John Thie, D.C., from California; and Sheldon Deal, D.C., from Tucson Arizona.

Here are four very powerful, yet very simple Touch For Health techniques you can use immediately on yourself or on others, often with astounding results. They only take ten to thirty seconds, but give incredible results!

ESR

ESR stands for Emotional Stress Release. As the neuro-vascular points for the Pectoralis Major Clavicular muscle associated with the stomach acupuncture meridian, these may be the most powerful and useful reflex points in Touch For Health. Because ESR is so simple, it is under estimated and under utilized. I have seen dramatic results hundreds of times in using ESR the last twenty years, especially for "erasing" or defusing trauma. People tend to use this technique instinctively when they are under stress or in a crisis. Now you can use this powerful technique consciously to help yourself and others in a dramatic way.

The ESR points are located on the Frontal Eminence, which

is directly above the center of each eye, about half way between the eye brow and hairline.

The technique involves simply holding these two points with the finger tips with a light touch (no more pressure than you'd put on your eyeball). If one hand is being used, the thumb can be used on one side; however, using both hands is more effective.

While holding these ESR points, think about the stress. Hold for ten seconds up to several minutes, depending on the severity of the stress. Focus on the stress and its source.

The stress can be emotional, particularly fear, anger and sadness or grief, and it can be from the past (recent or from childhood), in the present or in the future (anticipated).

The stress could also be physical, such as a headache, backache, or from an injury or accident. Most headaches can be eliminated within 10-20 seconds using ESR. Often pain in other areas of the body can be reduced or eliminated as well.

Having another person do ESR for you may be more effective than doing it on yourself.

Often you can tell that you've held the ESR points long enough when one of two things occur: you feel both pulses synchronize or the person takes a deep involuntary breath.

Even when you see no obvious results, there is a significant reduction of internal stress and trauma that can be demonstrated with kinesiological muscle testing.

The reason this works is because activating these ESR points stimulates the flow of blood in the brain from the posterior lobes to the frontal lobes, which helps you come out of a reactive mode (fear and anger) to a rational and creative mode of thinking.

I do this every evening as I lie in bed as a sort of clearing of the day, even if nothing stressful happened.

Energy "Reset" Points

The energy reset points are known as the K-27 reflex points. They are similar to a master circuit breaker that gets switched off when your body is under more stress than it can safely handle. It is like a safety or protection mechanism.

Also, when you are feeling overwhelmed with stress, one of the hemispheres of your brain will become overly dominant, which will disable the opposite side to an extent. This decreases "brain integration" which can manifest with dyslexic patterns such as reversing numbers or letters, fatigue, a lack of coordination and many other symptoms.

Even though your system will eventually "reset" by itself, you can immediately switch "the power" back on manually by simply rubbing these points for five to ten seconds. This involves simply vigorously rubbing the last acupuncture points (the "K-27's") on the Kidney acupuncture meridian. Even more effective is to shine a pointer laser for a couple seconds on these points instead of rubbing them.

They are located on your chest in the sternal notch, which is directly beneath the collar bone and next to your sternum. These points are about one inch from the midline of your chest, directly below your eyes. *For best results, hold one hand over your navel as you rub your K-27 points.* You can do both at the same time or one at a time which is what I prefer.

I take a few seconds to stimulate these points every morning just to enhance my brain integration and whenever I feel overwhelmed with stress, either from a crisis or just an accumulation of stuff. This is something that you can do before you even get out of bed! Try it.

Brain Integration

Cross crawling is another easy and fun way to reduce stress and enhance brain integration. Simply march in place, swinging your hands freely while you think of someone you appreciate. Make sure that the arm that moves up is opposite of the leg that you are lifting. You can also cross over and touch the opposite knee with your hand.

Do this for 10-20 seconds at least once a day, especially in the morning, and *anytime* you feel anxiety, pressure or stress.

Mental Acuity

The lymph system is the drainage system of the body. There are many neuro-lymphatic reflex points that regulate the energy to various parts of the lymphatic system. There is one set that is especially useful for regaining clear thinking or defusing "brain fog."

Massage for ten to thirty seconds the area from the bone at the front of the shoulder joint down along the outside of the breast on the side of the chest (about four inches).

Do the same for the posterior neuro-lymphatic points located just under the backside of your skull where it joins the neck, about 2-3 inches from the center line.

Improvement is usually instant and often dramatic. Many other neuro-lymphatic reflex points that relate to other organ functions are located between the ribs where they attach to the sternum in the middle of your chest in front or where they join the spine on your back. These to can be rubbed.

Hugs

Giving and receiving hugs is an excellent way to reduce stress, either during or better yet, as a preventative measure. The experts say we need twelve hugs a day to stay healthy.

"Freeze-Frame"

These next two are Heart Math techniques based on the amazing HeartMath technology. This is very powerful in defusing stress, especially in a crisis. There are five simple steps:

1. Recognize your feelings of stress and "freeze-frame" them as you would put your VCR on pause to freeze a particular frame.

2. Focus your attention on the area of your physical heart, and breathe *deeply*, pretending that you are breathing through your heart. Do not move your chest as you breathe. Instead, move your diaphragm muscle (it feels like you are moving your stomach) down as you inhale and relax. Breathe this way for ten seconds.

3. Recall a positive or happy time in your life and mentally put yourself back into that situation (re-experience it). Or better yet, think of someone you really appreciate, and feel that apprecia-

tion from your heart. Do this for at least ten seconds.

4. With your focus still on your heart, ask your heart (or ask God through your heart) what an alternative perspective you could have on this situation, and what response could you have that was more efficient or appropriate.

5. Listen to what you hear and act accordingly.

"Heart Lock-In"

Focus your attention on the area of your physical heart, and breathe deeply, pretending that you are breathing through your heart. Think of someone (i.e. your spouse, God, your best friend, etc.) you really appreciate, and feel that appreciation deeply from your heart.

Get the maximum benefit by doing this "Heart Lock-in" procedure for 15 minutes as you listen to Heart Zones music developed by HeartMath. If you do this for 15 minutes, the benefits will last for four hours.

For more information on HeartMath, go to www.heartmath.com or call (800) 700-1238.

{ 13 }

REVITALIZED WATER

We live in the information age. It is well known that information, in the form of frequencies, is carried on many mediums, including electro-magnetic waves (radio, TV, cell phones, etc.), light (fiber optics), metal wires and integrated circuits to name a few. Few people realize that water also is a carrier of information. As such, the damage to water is far more than the pollutants and toxic chemicals it contains; it is damaged by the information (frequencies) that it picks up from these pollutants. Simply removing the toxic chemicals by filtration or purification does *not* eliminate the harmful information still retained by the water.

A new technology was developed in Austria ten years ago that neutralizes the impact of pollutants by "erasing" the negative information and restoring the original positive information (frequencies) back to water. This remarkable "Grander Technology" effectively revitalizes water in a manner congruent with the principle of homeopathy, in which specific information is imprinted into a liquid to be used as a medical remedy. Sometimes referred to as "living water", this can be another important deposit into your health account.

Tap water can be revitalized either one glass at a time with a unit the size of a pen (at a cost of 24 cents a week over ten years), or the entire house can be done permanently with a device the size of a shoe box. The advantage of having all the water revitalized is the "softening" or "conditioning" effect without the use of chemicals.

For free information on this unique health enhancing technology, call (800) 234-1351 or (206) 938-5800.

{ 14 }
HOW TO BE A HERO INSTEAD OF A VICTIM

Have you ever saved someone's life? How do you imagine it would feel?

When I was a teenager, I took a course to be certified as a lifeguard. I vividly remember (as if it were yesterday) being at the Sandy River in Troutdale, Oregon, probably in 1969. I heard a young lady yelling for help. She had been swept away by the current, and was drowning. I quickly swam toward her, clearly remembering my instructor's stern warning that the rescuer can easily become a victim of a desperate drowning person if he/she grabbed you.

The young woman indeed tried to grab me. I was able to forcibly disengage and reattempt the rescue. I was able to properly secure her in a firm grip, with my arm around her chest exactly as I'd been taught. Slowly I swam to shore.

She was extremely grateful, and I felt fantastic to have saved the life of another human being!

How would *you feel* if you were able to be a hero and save a person's life?

What if there was a simple way to do exactly that on a regular basis?

What if you could be a hero, for not just one person, but for hundreds or thousands? *How would that feel?*

The greatest psychological need we each have as human beings is to affirm our value, importance and significance. This is most powerfully achieved when we make a significant contribution and a positive difference for another human being. Saving and changing lives qualifies!

I've made it my mission and life purpose to enrich and save lives with the information you have read in this book. I can't think of anything more meaningful and fulfilling than saving and changing lives. Many times I've wept with joy and amazement as I've listened to dramatic stories of people's lives being changed or even saved.

I invite you to join me and thousands of others already enrolled in this vital mission to help people. Millions are dying needlessly as victims, and you can be one of the heroes!

You don't need any experience or special skills. All you need is a love for people, a strong desire to make a difference, and a way to do it.

Three thousand years ago, a prophet said, *"My people perish for lack of knowledge."* By bringing this vitally important knowledge of the five strategies, you can save and change lives.

Here's an example of how easy it is to make a difference for a lot of people. What if you saw a great movie and told just four people about it and they saw it too. That wouldn't take any special skills would it? What if those four people liked it, and did exactly what you did within the next week, which could easily happen (it happens all the time, doesn't it)? Now four plus sixteen others have seen the movie, *because of your influence* through the first four people you told.

The third week, the sixteen each tell their four best friends, who also go to see the movie. Now it's up to sixty-four people.

If the pattern continues (everyone telling just four), by the fourth week, 256 more people will see the movie. The next week, it will be over a thousand people. The next week, it will be over four thousand people, then 16,000, etc.

Because of your influence on just four people, thousands of people could have their lives impacted in at least a small way. You wouldn't be a hero *in this example*, because the movie is not saving or changing lives.

This is precisely how Christianity or any religion spreads. This is how most businesses grow—people telling people.

But what if you used this multiplication dynamic to spread information that was more significant than seeing a great movie, or eating at an excellent restaurant?

Within a short time you could make a significant difference in the lives of thousands of people.

This simple and natural process has allowed me to indirectly make a meaningful difference in the lives of over 250,000 people in the last five years. There is absolutely no feeling in the world like knowing you are making a difference in saving and changing lives.

I invite you to join me on this exciting mission of sharing life changing health information, including your personal story. Your reward, both emotionally and financially is absolutely awesome!

{ 15 }

HOW TO GET ALL YOUR ESSENTIAL NUTRIENTS FOR FREE!

For this material to make sense, be sure that you have read the prior appendix section on "How to be a hero instead of a victim."

It's actually quite easy to get all your essential nutrients for free. All you have to do is decide that that is what you want to do, and then continue doing what you've been good at doing since you were a child: talk to people about what you are excited about and believe in. Everyone does this already. We all get a benefit from doing it—we feel good that we are passing on valuable information, which affirms our value and helps us feel important and significant.

At the same time, this normal and natural activity of recommending and promoting something is not usually an activity where you are paid in dollars—you get paid *emotionally* by feeling good about yourself because you are helping someone.

Some of the most important essential nutrients are available, not only at a wholesale price by simply registering with the company, but can be received essentially for "free." As you refer other people to the manufacturer, you can receive monthly "thank-you" checks for the referrals you've made to the company, based on their purchases. Within thirty to ninety days, these referral checks can equal or exceed your monthly "health investment," thereby making the products you consume "free."

Thousands of people have already done this, and are getting all their "life support" health products essentially for "free."

Many others, including myself, have discovered that this can be taken even further, to the point that the weekly and monthly "thank-you" checks not only exceed the cost of personal use products, but that it can exceed and replace one's normal source of income. It's worked for thousands of others—why not you? To hear a three minute recording on this exciting concept, call (888) 800-6369 Extension 1121.

{ 16 }

SOCIAL STATUS AND YOUR HEALTH

Thirty years of scientific research has established that the most powerful predictor of human disease is social and economic inequality.

In the past 5 years, 193 studies have been published on various aspects of socioeconomic status and health, according to the New York Times.

The National Institutes of Health last year declared the relationship between social status, race and health to be one of its top priorities.

As the <u>New York Times</u> reported June 1, 1999 in its weekly Science Section,

"Scientists have known for decades that poverty translates into higher rates of illness and mortality. But an explosion of research is demonstrating that social class — as measured not just by income but also by education and other markers of relative status — is one of the most powerful predictors of health, more powerful than genetics, exposure to carcinogens, even smoking."

"What matters is not simply whether a person is rich or poor, college educated or not. Rather, risk for a wide variety of diseases, including cardiovascular disease, diabetes, arthritis, infant mortality, many infectious diseases and some types of cancer, varies with RELATIVE wealth or poverty: the higher the rung on the socioeconomic ladder, the lower the risk."

It isn't the absolute level of well-being that matters so much as the relative level. Even among the well-to-do, those higher on the social scale are healthier.

As the <u>New York Times</u> put it, current research is showing that a mid-level executive in a three-bedroom home in Scarsdale, N.Y. is more vulnerable to illness than his boss who lives in a 5-bedroom home a few blocks away.

No one is yet sure how all the components of this problem fit together. A sense of control of one's life is a key part of it. Stress is another. Social exclusion and residential segregation — especially by race but also by class — have important negative impacts.

A sense of opportunity, dignity, self-esteem, the respect of others — all these are important for health.

Social cohesion — a sense of neighborliness — also plays a role: people live longer in places where they believe they can trust their neighbors.

As Harvard economist Juliet Schor says, *"The reasons may not turn out to be so very complicated. Humans are social. We judge our own situations very much in comparison to others around us. It is not surprising that people experience less stress, more peace of mind, and feel happier in an environment with more social cohesion and more equality."*

If relative standing in the community is what matters most in protecting public health, then the modern world has been headed in the wrong direction for at least 20 years. Inequality has been increasing for 20 years. Most households in the U.S. have lower net worth than they did in 1983, and the wealthy few are far wealthier than they were in 1983.

Between 1983 and 1995, the inflation-adjusted net worth of the top 1% of Americans swelled by 17% while the bottom 40% of households lost 80%. In other words, the gap between the rich and the poor has widened. *It is this widening gap that gives rise to disease, research shows.*

This problem is not restricted to the U.S., though the U.S. suffers from greater inequality than any other industrialized nation. The United Nations HUMAN DEVELOPMENT REPORT 1998 points out that in 100 countries, incomes today are lower in real terms than they were a decade ago.

Within the U.S., the gap between rich and poor is growing. Here is a list of some indicators:

** Shrinking wages. Despite some growth in wages in 1996 and 1997, hourly workers in 1998 still earned 6.2% less per hour (adjusted for inflation) than they did in 1973 when Richard Nixon was President.

** The median income of young families with children was 33% lower in 1994 than it was in 1973.

** The average worker worked 148 more hours in 1996 (1868 hours) than in 1973 (1720 hours). That's equivalent to nearly 4 weeks additional work each year, to make ends meet.

** For 20 years, companies have been withholding wages from workers and transferring that wealth to executives. In 1980, the average CEO in *Business Week's* annual survey made 42 times as much as a factory worker.[2,pg.32] By 1997, the average CEO was making 326 times as much as a factory worker.

** Pensions are slowly disappearing, and the quality of pension programs is rapidly declining. Only 47% of workers are covered by pension plans (down from 51% in 1979).

** Savings are a thing of the past. The U.S. personal savings rate has fallen from 8.6% in 1984 to 2.1% in 1997 and 0.5% in 1998. People are spending a larger portion of their incomes on health care, child care, housing, and college tuition.

** *The American Journal of Public Health* in 1998 reported that 10 million Americans — including more than four million children — do not have enough to eat; a majority are members of families with at least one member working.

The good news is that **you** don't have less health by being on the short end of the financial stick. Why not put yourself on the higher end of the spectrum by finding a solid business about which you can really be passionate? You can start your adventure part-time out of your home as I did (every day over 7000 people begin a home based business).

Why not, as you are improving your economic and social status, enjoy the automatic benefit of improving your health at the same time?

{ 17 }

HOW TO BE SUPREMELY HAPPY!

Everyone wants to be happy. In fact, your health is dependent on how happy you are. Happiness or joy is how you feel when you have a belief or perception that you are getting some kind of benefit, or something of value.

The greatest happiness occurs when you experience the greatest value or benefit. The higher the perceived value, the higher the level of happiness.

Where do we experience the greatest happiness? It is when we are being most strongly affirmed as an important, significant and valuable person.

The same five strategies to vibrant health, and longevity apply to creating the maximum experience of personal happiness. Let's start again with the Fire dynamic, which has to do with your heart.

The Happy Heart

Your heart is the way to happiness. Three thousand years ago, King Solomon wrote, "*Pay close attention to your heart, for from it flow the springs of life.*" (Proverbs 23)

Don't you feel happy when you are living from your heart, and feel passionate about something?

Don't you feel happy when you are on a mission to make a difference?

Don't you feel happy when you are loved and valued by another person? And the more important this person is in your eyes, the more you feel valued by this relationship.

What if this important person was God? What if you could experience the depth of infinite love that could only come from an infinite being? What if this love was not diminished by what you had done or not done? Can you see how that could be your wellspring of happiness?

What if you could be on a mission for God? Wouldn't you feel important and significant? What would that do for your happiness and fulfillment?

Wouldn't having a sense of purpose and destiny, and living from your heart with passion give you the greatest experience of happiness?

That's exactly what I have found. Here's how my step-son, John Day describes his experience of having a clear purpose in his relationship with God:

"*Three years ago, I was a passionate little punk. My purpose and dream in life was to play music, (punk rock), have fame, drugs and girls. I was very dedicated to writing songs, practicing with my band, making friends with the right people and being crazy enough to stick out of the crowd. I was on track to what I "thought" I wanted. In the fall of 1996, I found myself in a little grass hut in Western Samoa in a rehab program. I was at the end of my rope, and I surrendered my life to Jesus and became a Christian ("little Christ").*

"Some people think that to become a Christian you have to lose all of your "irreverent" qualities and begin to act like a monk—no fun, no adventure, no life. What I have found is that this is a complete lie!! God created all people the way they are for a reason and so all that I did was change my focus, not who I was. Now, with a clear purpose in life, I am passionate for Jesus. I live and breathe to do His will and I am on a mission to impact eternity. Now that I have fire in my heart, I am really happy.

"As for music, well God has called me to lead my generation in worship and praise of our King. Every day that I am on this planet I have a reason to live, something to accomplish, ground to take for the Kingdom of God. It is awesome! And I know that God has an incredible plan for everyone that is willing to surrender his/her life to Him. I don't need to try to control everything anymore—and I am finding myself living the most incredible life I could imagine. The most wonderful part though is simply getting to know Jesus, my King, my Creator, my best friend. Imagine me, a nineteen year old having conversations with the Creator of the universe every day. Wow! My life will never be the same now that I have a new purpose and passion. I encourage you to do find your purpose and passion in God so you can have the level of happiness I have!" **John Day**

What if you could experience God as a treasure chest of incalculable wealth?

This is exactly how Jesus described it: *"The kingdom of heaven is like a treasure hidden in a field, which a man found and hid; and from JOY (happiness) over it he goes and sells all that he has, and buys that field."* (Matthew 13:44)

Why not go for **maximum happiness** by letting God be the love of your life? Let Him fill your heart and life with Himself.

It is an exciting possibility, and it can be an awesome reality!

Being Well Connected

The Earth dynamic symbolizes being connected with another person. Wouldn't you agree that the happiest people in the world are those who are most intimately connected with another person?

What if there were a way to be intimately connected with the all powerful God of the universe, the One who cares about you more than any other human? What if you could experience a sense of intimate oneness that surpassed anything in human relationships? Wouldn't *that* make you feel valued? Wouldn't that make you feel happy and fulfilled?

Three thousand years age, King David wrote: *"In Your presence is fullness of joy, and at your right hand are pleasures forever!"* (Psalms 16:11)

My experience, and that of millions of others, is that the presence of God is absolutely real. I believe that it can be for you as well. Happiness can be found in many places in many different ways. But if you want **maximum happiness**, satisfaction and fulfillment, God is the only place (person) where it can be found, in being connected with Him as your loving Father.

Here's one way Jesus described being connected to God:

"I am the vine, you are the branches. When you are joined with me and I with you in an intimate and organic relationship, the harvest is sure to be abundant. Separated, you can't produce a thing. I've told you this for a reason: that my happiness might be your happiness, and your happiness be fully mature." John 15:5,11.

Just make sure you don't settle for the cheap counterfeit of "religion." Religion can be an empty and seductive substitute for the real thing. Why not reject religion and choose relationship with God?

To me, "religion" is trying to be good enough to be okay with

God, rather than having a personal connection and relationship with Him. I see religion as a deceptive form of bondage, whereas a relationship with God (knowing, trusting and loving Him) is life, happiness and freedom. It is also the best route to "life, liberty and the pursuit of happiness."

I used to be "religious." For years, I was a blind, but self-righteous and arrogant "Pharisee." Jesus spoke of this insidious religious mindset as he quotes Isaiah from about 700 years earlier: *"This people honor me with their lips, but their heart is far away from Me. Their "worship" is worthless."* (Isaiah 29:13 and Matthew 15:8)

I've found that whereas *religion* is empty, a *relationship* with the Father is full and satisfying, and my greatest source of happiness. Why not break the shackles of religion and experience the **maximum happiness** that can only be found in being connected with God in a personal relationship?

Here's my wife's experience of having a personal connection with God:

"With all the stress that life has to offer, happiness sometimes seems like an elusive butterfly. I wasn't surprised when I read an article on a study that had found that women experience more stress than men. Just think of all the societal and cultural expectations placed on women. It can be overwhelming! The majority of stress in my life comes from the multiplicity of roles I play: wife, mother, stepmother, daughter, sister, friend, hostess, etc, and the expectations related to each of them.

"The greatest stress reliever I've found is quite simply in my daily quiet time with God, and observing His handiwork in nature. As I read my Bible and meditate on what God is saying to me in His Word, I feel reconnected with God. I enjoy His precious presence and His love for me. And when I get out into nature for a walk, or look at an incredible sunset, or watch a hummingbird flitting around my flowerpots, I especially enjoy my sense of oneness with God. It's an incredible experience! Being intimately connected with the Almighty, All Powerful God puts all the stress I experience into a manageable perspective. A peace that surpasses understanding gracefully envelops me, and, I find myself at a new level of happiness!" I've tried many other ways to relieve stress, and

so many of these create a stress of their own. Truly, doing whatever I can to personally connect with the God who loves me is the best way I've found to relieve my stress and live a glorious life!" **Diana Gebauer**

Here's the experience of another person's connection with God:

"My happiness in God has been developed over 20 years of walking with Him. Even though I am made in His Image, there is an ongoing process of developing the character of Jesus Christ. This happens only as I stay connected as a branch needs to stay connected to the vine in order to have life. In my mid 20's, I found myself in the biggest trial of my life, and spent the midnight hours praying and seeking God. I was asking earnestly for God's help, saying "God, Help me get through this... help me get through this." The trials were so intense, I didn't know what else to pray.

"After months of travail concerning my trials, I finally surrendered and told the Lord that I would serve him and love him no matter what — even if the trial continued! All he wanted was my heart and my will. He turned my breakdown into a breakthrough, and I felt connected with God. He is so faithful! All the time I see Him work miracles through people, prayer, and dreams.

"I continue to experience the goodness of God beyond my expectations. I love to feel His presence. Jesus Christ, our perfect example always yielded to His heavenly Father and continually said "not my will but Thine be done." Like Jesus, I surrender my will to the Lord daily because I have learned that surrender to God is how I keep my connection with Him. This is the major key to my happiness." **Diane Petticord**

Foreign Invaders

The Metal dynamic symbolizes foreign toxins in the body. Toxins clearly interfere with health, life and eventually our happiness on the physical plane of existence. In the same way, "Spiritual toxins" interfere with our health, life, freedom and eventually our happiness on the spiritual level, where it counts the most.

What are "spiritual toxins?" These deadly invisible toxins include bitterness, anger, self-centeredness, fear, and hopeless-

ness, as well as the root toxins of pride, arrogance and self-righteousness. The inevitable result of these insidious toxins, also
known as sin, is death on any number of levels, including rela-
tional and spiritual ("the wages of sin is death"). Sin is any
thought, attitude or action that is based on pride, rebellion or
self-centeredness, as opposed to being based on trust, love and
living for God.

"Everyone who sins is the slave of sin." John 8:34

Do you like the idea of being a slave? Wouldn't you prefer to be
free of the spiritual toxins in your life, such as bitterness, anger,
self-centeredness, fear, hopelessness, pride, arrogance and self-
righteousness?

How do you get free of these fatal spiritual toxins? You can't—
at least on your own. But there is a way to freedom, and it is provided by the personal God of love through forgiveness. When
we repent for our sins *from our heart* (Fire dynamic), and ask for
forgiveness based on trust in God's provision through the death
of His Son, Jesus, as our substitute, we can be instantly cleansed
and forgiven as we receive the free gift of eternal life.

Here's the promise of freedom of which Jesus spoke: *"If you
hold to my word, you are truly disciples of mine; and you shall know the
truth, and the truth shall make you free. If the Son makes you free, you
will really be free."* John 8:31-32, 35

Going though this door of freedom opens you to the level of
maximum happiness that cannot be known in any other way.

Jesus put it this way: *"I am the door; if anyone enters through me,
he will be saved. I came that you might have life, and might have it
abundantly* (that is, to the max!)."

Here is a modern day testimonial that demonstrates this:

"I was born into a world of chaos and destruction. My parents were

violently divorced while I was still in the womb, and in my very DNA there was sin, death, and destruction. My mother remarried a man when I was 4 who was schizophrenic and extremely abusive. He created in me a deep fear that stole my very sense of innocence. I lived in complete fear that only got worse when my family tried to rescue me and I didn't see my Mom again for over 5 years, 5 years of hell with suicide beckoning me in and only fear keeping me alive. I tried to be a lover, but pain has a way of getting even to the most tender parts of your heart. My life continued in this downward spiral until I ended up alone, living in the gutters of America in and out of jail at the age of only 15.

"I didn't care and didn't feel a thing - a crusty punk on a mission to destroy the world with my bottle of booze. I was a lonely confused kid, and I thought that a religiously brainwashed society of selfish hypocrites was to blame. My heart was as hard as cement and I was enslaved to a wicked task master, SIN. My life was out of control. I would be dead, in jail, or worse today if it wasn't for the intervention of God.

"I was so lost that I blindly agreed to go 6,000 miles away to a reformatory boot camp on Tonga, a little island in the South Pacific. It was the freakiest place I had ever been and after 4 months of living hell I was about ready to throw it all in and give it all up. It was then that I learned of the amazing love of the Savior. I opened up a Bible that somebody sent me and it immediately pierced my innermost being, awakening my spirit and stirring my faith, hope and love. I learned of one who could give me a life of happiness free from the bondages of sin and death. I learned of sacrificial love of one who lived a sinless life and died an excruciating death, taking all my sin upon himself so that I could live a superabundant life and spend eternity with the greatest lover of all, Jesus Christ.

"It was then that I said "God, I am the dirtiest sinner in all of the world! But if you can use me here I am." Immediately, I experienced a whole new life, it was as if I was living for the first time ever. From that time on springs of joy have sprung forth from my heart, the rivers of living water, of the life and love of Jesus Christ. I have no greater joy than to know the love of God and call him Father. I had been lost and separated because of the blinding effect of sin, but now sin no longer has a

*hold on me and I am free to live a life of peace and happiness. I have
learned that the answer to my life was not in me trying to be a better person. It was when I admitted that I was weak and helpless, and allowed
God to take over my life that I was set free to live a life of an unshak-
able deep seated happiness.* Zachary Daly

Rushing Water

The Water dynamic represents movement. Movement is a sure
sign of life. A person may be moving physically, but if they are
not moving spiritually, they are "dead in the water."

When we are moving in and with God, we are happy and fulfilled. In His greatness and goodness, God is always on the
move, and He extends His gracious invitation to us to join Him
in what He is doing on His mission (*"Thy kingdom come, Thy will
be done, on earth as it is in heaven"*). When we are on a mission for
God, it can be like being Indiana Jones in the movie, *Raiders of
the Lost Ark.*

*Why settle for moving along with the crowd when you can be moving
with God?*

Life is like a race. If you just sit there, you lose. If you are going
to "run," why not run for the greatest prize? Why not run for God
and let Him reward you? God has rewards for us that are beyond
our wildest imagination. Talk about **maximum happiness!**

We are told to *"run the race set before us with endurance, laying
aside every encumbrance and the sin that so easily entangles us, fixing
our eyes on Jesus, the author and perfecter of faith."* (Hebrews 12:1-2)

Paul said it this way: *"Forgetting what lies behind, I <u>press on</u> toward
the goal for the prize of the upward call of God in Christ Jesus."* (Phil.
3:13-14) and *"<u>Run</u> in such a way that you may win."* (I Cor. 9:24)

Jesus said it this way: *"I am the light of the world; he who <u>follows</u> me
shall not <u>walk</u> in the darkness, but shall have the light of life."* (John 8:12)

When I choose to follow God, *"surely goodness and mercy will
<u>follow</u> me all the days of my life, and I will dwell in the house of the
Lord forever."* (Psalms 23:6)

Why not move with the One who is able to give you the greatest benefits and the **maximum happiness**, both in this life and in the one to come?

Here's the promise: *"Move toward God and He will move toward you."* (James 4:8-10)

Why not sign up for the real race of life? Why not run with God? The sign up fee for you has already been paid in full! It's free!

The way you "sign up" is by simply choosing to trust in God and love Him with all your heart, surrendering your life to Him, the Master coach.

It's the best decision I've ever made, and I highly recommend it to you. There are there immediate health benefits (physically, emotionally and spiritually), but the benefits literally go on forever, and the "retirement benefits" are out of this world!

Here's the experience of how one person moves with God:

"The greatest moments of happiness have been times I have been moving with God. When I am moving with someone, I am in harmony with them. It's like when I sang in a college quartet. When the voices completely harmonized there was a beautiful resonance. Now my life resonates with God. It is amazing that God offers Himself to us in that way. It's not always easy to be in harmony with God and move with Him. Sometimes it's easier to just do my own thing. But when I am walking with God, I enjoy a deep sense of intimacy and happiness, like a spring of fresh water bubbling up inside of me.

"One of the great chapters in my life was learning to move with God on the streets of San Francisco. I had a nightly television program in the Bay Area and mobilized churches to help the homeless and needy. We fed, clothed, and ministered many times to the homeless at Powell and Market streets. All that came and worked with us could feel a sense of God's moving with us and us with Him in partnership. God was certainly happy with what we were doing and we shared His pleasure.

Once you have experienced moving with God, you won't want to settle for anything less. You want it again and again. Adam "walked with God in the garden" and we were to walk with Him too. When I am moving with God as my best friend and co-pilot, my life takes on a new dimension of happiness." **Jerry Brandt**

"One of the greatest joys of my life was when God got a hold of me. I have been in full time ministry for over twenty years and have been in thirty six countries and I found my greatest happiness is walking into the flow of God and letting Him lead me into new places with Him. I always hungered for more of God from the time I was born-again, and I always wanted more. When I flow with God and let Him move with me, I see miracles and healings take place. God has moved me into the prophetic ministry and it has taken me almost around the world. I have had the privilege of ministering prophetically to thousands of people and I am still in awe watching the Holy Spirit touch lives. A few years ago I was hit with the Holy Laughter and my ministry has taken a brand new turn. I found that the greatest joy in flowing with God is in receiving what he has for me and then making sure that I pass it on. Ask Him yourself. He has much more for you. Dive into the living waters and swim with God!" Proverbs 18:4. **Fred Vance**

Pleasure out of this World!

The Wood dynamic represents nourishment. Even though food is primarily for the purpose of nourishment to sustain our life and health, it's greatest attraction is the potential for pleasure and enjoyment.

Wouldn't you agree that one of the greatest pleasures in life is eating delicious food? Don't we always prefer food that will give us the greatest pleasure, especially if it is supporting our health at the same time?

But there is a spiritual kind of food that can give us far greater pleasure and satisfaction than any physical food can! Here's how King David expressed it: *"O God, You are my God! I can't get enough of you! I've worked up such a hunger for You... My soul is satisfied with You as with a fantastic holiday meal. I tell everyone how happy I am with you!" Psalms 63:1, 5 (paraphrase).*

"You invite us to drink freely from your river of pleasure; Taste and see that the Lord is good." (Psalms 36:8; 34:8)

Jesus taught us to ask, *"Give us this day our daily bread."* But there is a food of a higher dimension that can give us far greater pleasure than any physical food. He also said, *"Do not work for the food which perishes, but for the food which endures to eternal life, which I will give you."* (John 6:27)

But this is the greatest promise: *"I am the bread of life. I am the living bread that comes down from heaven; if anyone eats of this bread, he shall live forever."* (John 6:48, 51)

Do you ever feel like you are alive physically, but dead on the inside? Does it ever seem like life is just a dead-end street?

Why settle for vibrant health and longevity in your body when you can also have it in the spiritual dimension?

Here's how one woman describes her heavenly pleasure.

"No telling where I would be today without God; nobody really knows. However, the words to a song that I wrote recently expresses it this way:

"God You're good! You've picked me up out of the miry clay,
Set my feet on the rock to stay,
Delivered me when I was down and out…
I have so much to shout about! God You're Good!"

"In my experience God has impacted my life beyond measure! He gave me peace of mind when I didn't know what peace was. I thought I knew what happiness was but found real happiness in my innermost being because of relationship with Him. I feel cherished, nurtured secure and complete.

"I exchanged hopelessness for hope. Once I was depressed and now I'm impressed with Him and life. And I have His provision to fulfill His

vision in my life! I have found that nothing in this world can compare with the love and freedom I have in my relationship with my God. I am satisfied, fulfilled and very happy." **Tina Shelley**

"Just recently, one of my family members sold his business for forty million dollars. To many people, this is a classic story of the American dream. A few months later I was in his stately home, looking into his son's open casket, an eighteen-year-old young man, the life of every party, a strapping middle linebacker who was the MVP and captain of his 5A High School football team. He had overdosed on heroin! What agony! What heartbreak! All of the illusions and facades of worldly success came tumbling down.

"My personal discovery and ongoing experience is that because God is my loving Father, His instructions to me in His Word are for my highest good and my highest levels of fulfillment and happiness in every area of my life. As my Creator and best friend, He knows how I tick; spiritually, physically, and emotionally. And you know what has really blown me away is that as my Father He wants me to have a blast. As his Son Jesus said, I want you to have life and that more abundantly!

"Feasting on God's Word daily, and getting to know Him in a tangible, intimate way is my source of true nourishment and life. He Himself is my "daily bread." I have found that what Jesus said is absolutely true, that, "Man does not live by bread alone, but by every word that proceeds out of the mouth of God." I have found that there is no authentic success or fulfillment without His Son Jesus, and a life surrendered to Him and His Word." **Wesley Tullis**

Can I ask you a very important question? If you were to die today, do you know where you would go? Do you know with absolute confidence that it would be a place of happiness with God?

If you were to suddenly find yourself before God's throne of judgment (as I believe we all will someday), and He asked you *"Why should I let you spend eternity with Me?"* what would you say?

Would you say something about how you lived a good life? How do you know that your "good" would be good enough (it isn't)? How about the times when you weren't good?

You don't need to take a chance on something this important! You don't need to wonder or hope! *Today,* you can have a far greater experience of happiness (**maximum happiness**), AND absolute confidence that you can be happy forever! How? By simply, from your heart, trusting in God's Son, Jesus, as your Lord and Savior, the one who died in your place for your sins and rose again.

Make the switch from depending on yourself to depending upon Him.

By surrendering your life to the Father who loves you more than you can understand, you can have a far greater life of happiness and fulfillment both now and forever.

Read the words of Jesus:

*"I have told you these things for a <u>purpose</u>: that My happiness might be your happiness, and that your happiness may be wholly mature (made full or **maximized**)"* John 15:11.

Here is a beautiful story that may touch your heart in such a way as to shift your perspective and even change your life:

A wealthy man and his son collected rare works of art. They had everything in their collection, from Picasso to Raphael. They would often sit together and admire the great works of art.

When the Vietnam conflict broke out, the son went to war. He was very courageous and died in battle while rescuing another soldier. The father was notified and grieved deeply for his only son.

About a month later, just before Christmas, there was a knock at the door. A young man stood at the door with a large package in his hands He said, "Sir, you don't know me, but I am the soldier for whom your son gave his life. He saved many lives that day, and he was carrying me to safety when a bullet struck him in the heart and he died instantly. He often talked about you, and your love for art.

The young man held out his package. "I know this isn't much. I'm not really a great artist, but I think your son would have wanted you to have this."

The father opened the package. It was a portrait of his son, painted by the young man. He stared in awe at the way the soldier had captured the personality of his son in the painting. The father was so drawn to the eyes that his own eyes welled up with tears. He thanked the young man and offered to pay him for the picture.

"Oh, no sir, I could never repay what your son did for me. It's a gift."

The father hung the portrait over his mantle. Every time visitors came to his home he took them to see the portrait of his son before he showed them any of the other great works he had collected.

The man died a few months later. There was to be a great auction of his paintings. Many influential people gathered, excited over seeing the great paintings and having an opportunity to purchase one for their collection.

On the platform sat the painting of the son. The auctioneer pounded his gavel. *"We will start the bidding with this picture of the son. Who will bid for this picture?"* There was silence. Then a voice in the back of the room shouted. *"We want to see the famous paintings. Skip this one."*

But the auctioneer persisted. *"Will someone bid for this painting? Who will start the bidding? $100, $200?"* Another voice shouted angrily. *"We didn't come to see this painting...we came to see the Van Goghs, the Rembrandts. Get on with the real bids!"* But still the auctioneer continued. *"The son! The son! Who'll take the son?"*

Finally, a voice came from the very back of the room. It was the long-time gardener of the man and his son. *"I'll give $10 for the painting."*

Being a poor man, it was all he could afford. *"We have $10, who will bid $20?"*

"Give it to him for $10. Let's see the masters."

"$10 is the bid, won't someone bid $20?" The crowd was becoming angry. They didn't want the picture of the son. They wanted the more worthy investments for their collections. The auctioneer pounded the gavel. *"Going once, twice, SOLD for $10!"*

A man sitting on the second row shouted. *"Now let's get on with the collection!"*

The auctioneer laid down his gavel. *"I'm sorry, the auction is over."*

"What about the paintings?" they demanded angrily.

"I am sorry. When I was called to conduct this auction, I was told

of a secret stipulation in the will. I was not allowed to reveal that stipulation until this time. Only the painting of the son would be auctioned. Whoever bought that painting would inherit the entire estate, including the paintings. The man who took the son gets everything!"

God gave His son 2,000 years ago to die on a cruel cross. Much like the auctioneer, His message today is, "The son, the son, who'll take the son?" Because, you see, whoever takes the Son gets everything.

Author — Unknown

For more information on how you can have **maximum happiness** in this life, and how you can have absolute confidence about your spiritual health and your eternal destiny, call my friend Jerry Brandt or his wife, Mariana at (813) 814-0675, or CBN National Counseling Center at (800) 759-0700.

The classic book on happiness from a Biblical perspective is *Desiring God—The Confessions of a Christian Hedonist* by John Piper. This book has influenced my life more than any other book besides the Bible.

One of the most amazing and exciting videos I have ever seen is called **Transformations.** This "must see" video is absolutely astounding. I was stunned and inspired by it, and you probably will be too. It documents four *entire cities* (in South and Central America, Africa and California) that have been totally transformed socially and economically because of God. You will see that transformation is not meant to be limited to individuals—it is meant to transform entire communities. And it could even happen in *your city*. Call (800) 668-5657 to order this paradigm shifting video!

{ 18 }

MY PERSONAL INVITATION TO YOU—

Join our Freedom Crusade to Impact Lives All Around the World

Dear Fellow Human Being,

Over 95 percent of the American population are needlessly suffering and dying prematurely, and I am on a mission to do my part to change that. I am on a mission to *"...bring good news to the afflicted; ... bind up the broken-hearted, proclaim freedom to captives...and announce a time of healing (grace)."* My intention is to play my role in saving and changing the lives of people around the world.

I am inviting you to join me and the thousands of others already on this freedom crusade so that together we can give, as a precious gift of life, health freedom (vibrant health, happiness and longevity) to others.

Together we can make a HUGE difference for people, starting with *you* and *your* family, *your* city, and *your* country, as well as around the world. PLUS, in the process, in ways you can not yet even imagine, your life can be totally changed!

You already know that nothing is more fulfilling and rewarding than helping someone in a significant way. This is especially true when you dramatically change the course of just one person's life or even save a life. You feel like a hero! And if you can impact a lot of lives, you can feel like a "super hero"!

What if I could show you how to <u>feel like a hero everyday</u>, AND earn a decent income at the same time in exchange for helping change lives?

Six years ago, I was broke and desperate. I was looking and praying for any legal way to just make a decent income, ideally by working with and helping people. My prayer was answered in February 1994. Today, I am in the blessed and uncommon position that I don't need any more money and I don't even need to work. With God's help, I have achieved the dream of freedom— freedom of health, time and money, AND so have many of my friends. In this position, I am *free* to keep doing what I really enjoy most: making a meaningful difference for people around the world. *Now I am increasing my reach to even more people by getting this book into the hands of at least a million people in the next two years.* Of course I know I can't do it by myself. That's why I am asking you to join me. Even though I already have an "army" of over 250,000 people throughout America, Canada, Australia, the United Kingdom and Japan, this is not enough. It is just a small beginning to what we can all do together. I am requesting your help by joining us, and as a bonus, if you are interested, you can be compensated quite well for your involvement and contribution.

Why not be a part of this exciting mission to help save millions of lives, and as a natural consequence, earn an income (part-time or full time) in the process just as I have. If you join me in this cause, I promise you that your life will be enriched in ways you never expected, but specifically in four exciting ways:

1. Fulfillment

We feel fulfilled when what we do makes a meaningful difference, and especially when we feel we are making a valuable contribution into the lives of others. But to be totally honest with you, six years ago, this was not what I was thinking about—my focus was to make enough money to survive. It's amazing how much things can change in a few years! Now, my sense of fulfillment comes from being on a mission! Your contribution into the lives of others is more than a gift; it will powerfully affirm that you *are* an important valuable person, and greatly reduce the universal human fear that we are worthless and insignificant, that we are not good enough. You can *experience* the reality that you ARE somebody. Your contribution as an important member of my freedom team will affirm and consolidate your personal sense of value and worth.

2. Fun

When you are involved in changing people's lives, you will discover quickly that there is nothing more exciting and fun than being involved in helping people! YOU REALLY SHOULD LOVE WHAT YOU DO! This really is possible! Joining this freedom mission can be your ultimate adventure of a lifetime. I've heard thousands of people say exactly that, and you might as well discover it for yourself! Plus you can enjoy the sense of belonging to an extended family where you can be respected, nurtured and supported.

3. Financial

If you are interested in this part and have financial needs, you can benefit financially starting *immediately!* Your financial reward can start small and then snowball from $300 to $1000 dollars a month part time, to $3000 to $5000 a month full time, to as much as $100,000 and more per year. The company I work with has already paid out over $200,000,000.00 (two hundred million dollars) in the last few years to regular people like you and me! Why not get paid really well for helping people? Isn't it about time you caught up and got ahead? Isn't it time you got aboard a vehicle that can actually take you where you want to go in your life? Aren't you tired of empty promises and hype? Why not join thousands of those who have already achieved their dreams? You can too. Now it's *your* turn.

4. Freedom

This is the best part. *Money is a cruel joke without freedom to enjoy life.* Freedom is precious. People are willing to die for freedom. America was founded over this issue. Did you see the movies, <u>Braveheart</u>, <u>Prince of Egypt</u> and <u>The Matrix</u>? They were about *FREEDOM! But in our culture where we have our basic freedoms secured, the full <u>enjoyment</u> of freedom is elusive without sufficient money.*

Within one to four years, you can experience a new level of personal freedom just as many of my friends and I have.

This includes <u>time freedom</u>, which means spending your time doing what *you* enjoy most, *when* you want to do it, and more time for family and fun.

This also includes <u>lifestyle freedom</u>, which means you will be <u>free</u> to pursue all your dreams and secret desires without being held back by a lack of money, resources and time. Others have done it—why not you?

I went from living in someone's unfinished basement to owning a lake front dream house right on Lake Sammamish in beautiful Bellevue Washington. I'm FREE to live wherever I want. I'm FREE to travel anywhere and anytime I want. I'm totally FREE to do and *be* everything that God has intended for me to be. *How FREE do YOU want to be?*

Exactly What Would You Be Doing?

You will just keep doing exactly what you've been doing your entire life! And it's something you're already good at: simply talking to people about the things you believe in.

What do you normally do when you discover something you are excited about? You tell someone about it! Why? <u>Because you feel good about yourself</u> when you pass on information of interest or value! This is NOT selling—it is simply sharing from your heart how you feel and what you know. In fact, doing this affirms your inherent personal value when you are giving people information that helps them.

The inevitable result is that people appreciate you more when you give them valuable information.

This information could be about a new movie, a super sale at your favorite department store, an outstanding restaurant or your church, and people appreciate it, and they appreciate you caring enough to take the time to share.

It could just as easily be this book you are talking about.

It can just as easily be about the essential nutrients described in chapter seven.

Everyone's doing it already—it's called *referral marketing, trust marketing* or word of mouth advertising. All it is, is simply recommending what you believe in.

Instead of settling for just feeling good when you share valuable information, why not let someone pay you if they are willing to? Why work for free if someone is willing to pay you for it? You and everyone you know are *already* recommending and promoting something, but very few people get paid for doing this.

If you are providing a valuable service by giving out valuable information, *shouldn't* you get paid for it? Don't the teachers who provide the valuable service of teaching our children deserve and get more than just an emotional pay off of feeling good because the are making a contribution into the lives of children?

How Hard Do You Want To Play?

How hard you play depends on how big you want to win! And winning includes both the impact you make on people as well as the money you put in your pocket.

The easiest way to start is by recommending this book and the web site, www.cureanydisease.com, and talking about some of the ideas in it that impressed you the most. This book can be a very thoughtful and caring gift, and you can just tell everyone about it as you would about anything else you believe in. To support you in this, I will allow you to buy these books by the case at a special price of 70 percent discount (book stores usually get a 40-50 percent discount). Then you can give them away, resell them or loan them out. Just call (888) 882-8949.

When people want to know how to get the essential nutrients or effective weight loss products, you'll give them a toll free number through which they can buy them direct from the company at either retail or at wholesale. <u>Anyone can register for free</u> with the company with a single purchase (at wholesale) of any product they carry.

People will discover how easy it is to get their products for "free" by doing what you just did. Just spread the good news of how to have vibrant health and longevity. It only takes four who bring in four, and not only can you have "free" products within 30-90 days, you are moving rapidly toward an extra income of $300 to $1000 a month.

Because you are paid for your referrals to the company, the more you talk to people, the more money you earn. It's easy and it's fun! And as they talk to people they know, and they talk to people they know and so on and so on, you'll be getting paid on *multiple* generations, which means your income can grow exponentially as "your organization" does.

This way you are not *limited* to getting paid for just 8-10 hours a day on just your own work. You can get paid for a hundred or even a thousand hours a day or more!

How is this possible? You are paid based on the efforts of others, just as the president of a company earns income from the efforts of his employees, or a principal of a school is paid based on supporting the work of the teachers who teach the children!

Here's a simple example of how this can work for you. Let's say you talk to only one or two people a week about this book or these principles of health (we'll show you how to do this). Of these one or two people each week, only one PER MONTH decides to join you and do the same thing you are doing. If you do this every month for one year, and the people who join do the same thing (not all of them will), your income can be $5000 to $10,000 a month within twelve months. Or it may take longer, but after four years of doing this consistently and having fun in the process, you could very possibly be able to "retire" with an annual income of $100,000 or more.

I have many personal friends who have done exactly that, such as Steve and Tina Shelley, Mark Petticord, Don Partridge, Donna

Davis, Rich Cox, Fred Vance, Dr. Rod Milne, Dr. Steve Hines, Marcia Smith and many others. These are just a few of the people who have done that in <u>less</u> than four years—why not you?

This is EXACTLY what happened to me when I started. My first year I earned over $100,000 (I put in a lot of time), and now it's several times that. The reason my income is so high is because the more people I am impacting, *even indirectly*, the more money I earn. In fact, I'm still getting paid for what I did my first month over five years ago!

At first, I didn't know what I was doing, but I just talked to everyone because I was so excited with what I'd discovered! In fact, I felt a moral obligation to share this valuable life changing information.

It was obvious to me that this was either too good to be true, or too good to miss!

In the same way I got all the training and support I needed, you can too. Someone will be excited to "partner" with you and give you all the personal support and training you need to get you to whatever level of freedom you want (health, time or financial), as slow or fast as you want!

It's up to you to decide—*how free do you want to be?*

How serious are you about making a difference in the world?

How many people do you want to help in your lifetime?

Are ready to join me in my mission?

What's Your First Step?

Thank the person who did you the favor of giving, loaning or telling you about this book. Ask for information as to your next step. I promise that you will be excited about what you learn. In fact, once you begin to understand and see the whole picture, you may be so excited that you won't be able to get to sleep tonight!

If you discovered this book on your own and have no one to talk to, and do want to talk to someone, then contact my office at health@nwlink.com or Linda Martin at (888) 882-8949. We can direct you to someone who can work with you and give you all the answers, support and training you need to help you fully experience all the Fulfillment, Fun and Freedom you want.

Thank you in advance for considering joining me in my mission. I appreciate who you are and the contribution you will be making as a member of my team. I promise you, your future will be exciting, and you can be rewarded extremely well financially, as you find the fulfillment, fun and FREEDOM you've always dreamed about!

As I help you get what you want in your life, you will be helping me get what I want: to fulfill my vision of reaching millions of people around the globe with vibrant health, happiness and longevity!

Sincerely,

Ray Gebauer, "Man on a Mission"

P.S. This is a true *triple* win situation. **You** win because you'll be getting your health freedom for "free" and more personal freedom and fulfillment as you make as much money as you want.

The **world** wins too because people you influence (directly and indirectly) will have their lives changed.

I win because with your participation, I will be a step closer to fulfilling my mission of making a difference for more people around the world!

What could be better than a triple win of this magnitude!

P.P.S. If you can't wait to talk to a live person, you can call these toll free numbers 24 hours a day to hear your choice of several informative recorded messages:

(888) 800- 6339 Extension 1121   (3 minute message)
(888) 346-INFO (4636)   (10 options)

P.P.P.S. For a FREE GIFT of my WELLdisk ($10 value) that is an interactive health guide that gives you five simple free health tests and additional information, visit my web site listed below, or request a WELLdisk for free by calling (888) 666-8942 or (800) 700-1238. You can use both the WELLdisk (which can be emailed as an attachment) and the web site to easily introduce your friends to the five strategies for vibrant health, happiness and longevity you've learned in this book.

I wish for you the best of health—physically, emotionally, financially and spiritually.

www.cureanydisease.com
Health@nwlink.com

Resources

Here are some valuable resources to help you in achieving vibrant health, happiness and longevity. Most of these items were mentioned in the book, but for your convenience, they all are listed here. They are available by calling (800) 700-1238 (Washington) or (888) 666-8942 (Oregon). Shipping will be added to any order.

Books:

1. How to Cure and Prevent Any Disease by Ray Gebauer. (www.cureanydisease.com or (800) 700-1238 or (888) 666-8942)

Soft Cover or as an Audio Book
- By the Case—70 percent discount off the retail price ($25): **call (888) 882-8949** (10 cases—75 percent discount; 100 cases—80 percent discount)
- Three or more—60 percent discount ($30 for three).
- One or two—40 percent discount ($15 each).

Electronic Version of How to Cure and Prevent Any Disease
Three or more—60 percent discount off $10 retail price ($4 each)
One or two—40 percent discount ($6 each)

2. Unstoppable by Cynthia Kersey (45 inspiring stories)
3. Living With Passion – 10 Simple secrets That Guarantee Your Success by Peter Hirsch
4. The Joyful Spirit – How to Become the Happiest Person You Know by Brian Biro
5. Get A Life – How to Leave That Dead-End Job Behind and Create Your Perfect Future – Today! by Philip Stills
6. Mach II With Your Hair On Fire by Richard Brooke (my favorite book on developing a personal vision and self-motivation).
7. Freeze-Frame by Doc Childre (on HeartMath technology)
8. Your Body Knows Best by Ann Louise Gittleman (on health)
9. Becoming a Person of Influence by John Maxwell (on developing leadership)
10. What the Bible Says about Healthy Living by Russell, MD

FREE Audio Cassette Tapes:
(888) 666-8942 or (800) 700-1238 (small S/H charge)

1. The Nugent Report – Dr. Steve Nugent interviews Doctors on Glyconutrients
2. Confessions of a Heretic by Dr. Michael Schlachter, MD
3. GlycoLEAN—Lean Body System by Dr. Steve Nugent on effective weight loss
4. A Transformation in Health Care by Steve Lemme (Very educational)
5. Conspiracy Against our Children by Dr. Gemmer (about Ritalin)
6. Iceberg Ahead by Dr. Gemmer (Causes of the health crisis)
7. Mannatech—A Company of Destiny (A Spiritual Perspective) by Sam Caster
8. Acupuncture and Micro-Current and Health by Jim Suzuki (inventor) on the use of Bio-Therapeutic Computers (800) 234-0836

Web sites:

www.clickwell.com High quality generic supplements

www.glycoscience.com Published scientific articles on glyconutrients

www.drugawareness.org : For more information on the risk of using drugs

www.aicr.org : American Institute for Cancer Research

www.touch4health.com, www.tfh.org or www.kinesiology.net Kinesiology information

www.bridgequestinc.com or request a free Web-Disk by calling (800) 449-9488

www.touchstarpro.com/wellness.html How to customize humor to get maximum health benefits

www.dorway.com,www.presidiotex.com/aspartame, www.web2.airmail.net/marystod for shocking information on artificial sweeteners

www.notmilk.com or www.antidairycoalition.com see the documentation on the serious problems and misinformation on dairy products.

www.glycemic.com or www.mendosa.com/gilists.htm extensive information on glycemic indexing of foods

www.callpne.com Pharmacist Health Network for professional guidance on supplements and/or drug interaction. For scheduling a phone

appointment call 888-388-5522 or 900-CALLPNE
www.beeson.org/Livingto100/quiz.htm Take the actual test for FREE
with an instant calculation of your longevity
www.heartmath.com HeartMath technology
www.cureanydisease.com A free interactive health guide

Phone numbers:

Freedom Message: (888) 800- 6339 Extension 1121 – Three minute
recorded message on the five levels of Freedom
Information Line: (888) 346-INFO (4636) – Ten recorded messages on
glyconutrients and opportunity
Touch For Health Association at (800) 466-8342 (classes and information)
CBN National Counseling Center at (800) 759-0700 (For prayer or
counseling)
Action Evangelism: Jerry Brandt at jbrandt4him@hotmail.com or
(813) 814-0675 for spiritual counsel
Revitalized Water information (800) 234-1351 or (206) 938-5800
Bridgequest Inc. (800) 449-9488 (Personal development programs by
Mike Smith)

Miscellaneous:

Free brochure "Taking a Closer Look at Phytochemicals—New
Cancer Research" from the American Institute for Cancer Research
at (800) 843-8114
Free sample of flaxseed oil: (800) 445-3529 or visit www.barleans.com
WELLdisk –An Interactive Health Guide based on this book (**Free** at
www.cureanydisease.com or call 888-666-8942)
Vision—The Process of Passing it On by John Maxwell (An
incredible tape Album)
Take Charge of Your Life by Jim Rohn (Fantastic tape album)
My Story Workshop on tape by Jerry Brandt at jbrandt4him@hotmail.com,
www.actionevangelism.com or (877) 771-1319
Transformations Video (800) 668-5657
How Much Freedom Do You Want? Video (17 minutes) on how to
have all five levels of freedom in your life. (888) 666-8942 or
(800) 700-1238

Bibliography

Batmanghelidj, MD: Your Body's Many Cries for Water. Falls Church, Virginia: Global Health Solutions, Inc., 1995.

Biro, B: Beyond Success. Montana: Pygmalion Press, 1997.

Budwig, J: Flax Oil as a True Aid against Arthritis, Heart Infarction, Cancer and other Diseases. Vancouver, British Columbia, CANADA: Apple Publishing.

Burton Goldberg Group: Alternative Medicine. Puyallup, Washington: Future Medicine Publishing, 1993.

Carter, A: The Cancer Answer. Scottsdale, Arizona: A.L.M. Publishers, 1988. The New Miracles of Rebound Exercise. Scottsdale, Arizona: A.L.M. Publishers, 1988

Childre, Doc: Freeze Frame. Boulder Creek, California: Planetary Publications, 1998.

Chopra, MD: Ageless Body, Timeless Mind. New York: Harmony Books, 1993.

Deal, DC, NMD, DIBAK: Advanced Kinesiology. Tucson, Arizona: New Life Publishing Co. 1999

DeCava, MS, LNC: The Real Truth about Vitamins and Antioxidants. Columbus, Georgia: Brentwood Academic Press, 1996. Diamond, MD: Behavioral Kinesiology. New York: Harper & Row, 1979.

DeCava, MS, LNC: Cholesterol Facts and Fantasies. What Do the Experts REALLY Say? Centerville, Massachusetts: Printery, 1994.

Evans, PhD and Rosenberg, MD: Biomarkers—The Ten Keys to Prolonging Vitality: New York: Simon & Schuster, 1991.

Fischer, W: How to Fight Cancer & Win. Canfield, Ohio: Fischer Publishing Corporation, 1987.

Gittleman, MS, CNS: How to Stay Young and Healthy in a Toxic World. Los Angeles, California: Keats Publishing, 1999.

Gittleman, MS: Your Body Knows Best. New York: Simon & Schuster, 1997.

Hirsch, P: Living with Passion. Charlottesville, Virginia: MLM Publishing, 1994.

Kersey, C: Unstoppable. Naperville, Illinois: Sourcebooks, Inc., 1998.

Kelder, P: Ancient Secret of the Fountain of Youth. Gig Harbor, Washington: Harbor Press, Inc., 1985.

Maxwell, J: Becoming a Person of Influence. Nashville, Tennessee: Thomas Nelson Publishers, 1997.

Maxwell, J: Living at the Next Level. Nashville, Tennessee: Thomas Nelson Publishers, 1996.

Moore, N: The Facts about Phytochemicals. Dallas, Texas: Charis Publishing Co., 1996.

Morehouse, PhD and Gross, L: Total Fitness in 30 Minutes a Week. New York: Simon & Schuster, 1975.

Null, G: Reverse the Aging Process Naturally. New York: Villard Books, 1996.

Piper, J: Desiring God. Portland, Oregon: Multnomah Press, 1986.

Price, MD: Coronaries/Cholesterol/Chlorine. New York: Alta Enterprises, Inc., 1969.

Price, DDS: Nutrition and Physical Degeneration. La Mesa, California: The Price-Pottenger Nutrition Foundation, Inc., 1970.

Russell, MD: What the Bible Says about Healthy Living. Ventura, California: Regal Books, 1996.

Stills, P: Get a Life. Charlottesville, Virginia: Upline Press, 1995.

Thie, DC: Touch for Health. Marina del Rey, California: DeVorss & Company, Publisher, 1996.

Topping, PhD: Stress Release. Bellingham, Washington: Topping International Institute, 1985.

West, DN, ND: The Golden Seven Plus One. Orem, Utah: Samuel Publishing Company, 1981.